CHINA HANDBOO

SPORTS AND PUBLIC HEALTH

Compiled by
the *China Handbook* Editorial Committee
Translated by
Wen Botang

FOREIGN LANGUAGES PRESS BEIJING

First Edition 1983

ISBN 0-8351-0990-9

Published by the Foreign Languages Press
24 Baiwanzhuang Road, Beijing, China

Printed by the Foreign Languages Printing House
19 West Chegongzhuang Road, Beijing, China

Distributed by China Publications Centre (Guoji Shudian)
P.O. Box 399, Beijing, China

Printed in the People's Republic of China

EDITOR'S NOTE

More than 30 years have elapsed since the birth of the People's Republic of China on October 1, 1949. "How, really, is China today?" many people abroad wish to know. To answer this question, we plan to compile and publish a voluminous *China Handbook*, in which we intend to introduce the New China in every field of its activities. Emphasis will be on the process of development during the past three decades, the accomplishments, and the problems that still remain. The book will contain accurate statistics and related materials, all of which will be ready references for an interested reader.

To enhance the usefulness of the forthcoming volume, we plan to publish 10 major sections separately at first, so that we shall have an opportunity to take into consideration the opinions of our readers before all the composite parts are put together, revised and published as one volume. These separate sections are:

Geography
History
Politics
Economy
Education and Science
Literature and Art
Sports and Public Health
Culture

Life and Lifestyle
Tourism

Here, we wish particularly to point out the following:

First, the statistics listed in each separate book exclude those of Taiwan, unless otherwise indicated.

Second, the statistics are those compiled up to the end of 1980.

The *China Handbook* Editorial Committee

CONTENTS

Chapter One

SPORTS

1. DEVELOPMENT OF PHYSICAL CULTURE AND SPORTS IN NEW CHINA

Sports in old China — to the extent they existed — were the domain of the wealthy while most people suffered from poor health, making the metaphor applied to the whole Chinese people of the time, "the sickmen of East Asia". In competitive sports, not one Chinese name can be found among top world class athletes or world record holders of that era.

The founding of the People's Republic of China in 1949 brought fundamental changes to sports as it did to all aspects of Chinese culture. And in New China, as the old physical education systems were reformed into those which serve the people, the foundation was quickly laid for China to develop into a powerful country in sports. Today millions of people take part in physical training through regular programmes in schools, factories, communes, army units, government offices, etc. and in specialized training programmes and institutions. By 1956, New China was able to produce its first world record holder — Chen Jingkai in weightlifting, who became the forerunner of some 10 million title-holding sportsmen (including some 5,000 Chinese "Masters of Sports") who have broken over 200 world records and won 57 world championship titles. With general participation in sports activities throughout the country and with a fine contingent of Chinese sports men and women competing in all international games, the "sickmen of East Asia" have returned to good health.

From the beginning, the Chinese Communist Party and the government recognized the importance of physical culture and sports by adopting a series of measures to foster their sound development. Immediately after the founding of the People's Republic, the Party Central Committee issued a directive on "Strengthening the Work in Physical Culture and Sports for the People", and Chairman Mao Zedong wrote the inscription: "Promote physical culture; build up the people's health." Agencies were established at various levels, guiding policies set, and construction begun on sports facilities.

The encouragement of general participation in organized physical activities — including callisthenics, outdoor games, chess, the martial arts as well as other competitive sports — first of all improved the health standards for both the urban and rural populations. Among the new policies was a provision that office workers take two 10-minute breaks, in the morning and afternoon, for limbering-up exercises. Today with physical education an integral part of school curricula, more than 80 million young people and children have tested at the physical standard for their grade and age group.

The importance given athletic training is also shown in the establishment of 11 physical education institutes which over the years have turned out 28,000 graduates, and in the setting up of physical education departments in more than 110 teachers' colleges which have trained a large number of physical education teachers. These have been joined by a number of national and regional physical culture research institutes now engaged in scientific research in physical education and training. The government has also financed the construction of stadiums and gymnasiums all over the country.

The increased number of sports facilities and general raising of physical education standards consequently raised the level of performance in competitive sports. In 1953, Wu Chuanyu became the first Chinese swimmer to win a gold medal in an international competition. In 1959, Rong Guotuan brought home to China its first international title by taking the men's singles at the 25th World Table Tennis Championships. After Chinese sportsmen in the mid-1950s had, as one newspaper described it, broken the "big duck's egg" — "0" — in international competition, they were followed through the barrier by an ever-increasing number of athletes bringing credit to the Chinese people. By 1966, over 100 Chinese athletes had broken world records in weightlifting, archery, shooting, track and field events, swimming, parachute jumping, model aeroplane competition, speed skating, mountaineering, etc. In the process, 15 of these athletes won 13 world titles. Another big event of the sixties was the first successful ascent up the northern slope of Mount Qomolangma, the world's highest peak, by a Chinese mountain climbing team.

Unfortunately during the period of the "cultural revolution" from 1966 to 1976 the advance of sports in China was brought to a standstill as the two counter-revolutionary cliques of Lin Biao and Jiang Qing tried to negate every achievement in sports and physical education since the founding of New China. Athletes were persecuted, sports organizations immobilized, and facilities wrecked. The best years of many fine athletes were wasted, and many workers in the field of sports became victims of wanton persecution. The disruption of what had been a vigorously developing public sports programme brought about a drastic reduction in skills. The gap between Chinese and world standards in some items, which had been narrowed, widened again.

However after the fall of the Jiang Qing counter-revolutionary clique in October 1976, the Party and government worked hard to bring order out of chaos, and athletics recovered in less time than expected to make new headway. Policies for sports work became more flexible, opening even broader vistas in sports. New sports organizations were created and old ones reorganized on a sound basis; physical training and sports in schools resumed under improved standards; and sports activities among workers and peasants again assumed their vital role. Meanwhile, people began to organize themselves in all kinds of sports activities as the popularity of sports boomed. This included traditional sports such as *wushu* (martial arts) which began to be taken up by more and more people who recognized their value in promoting the health of the body and mind. Different *wushu* schools carried on the old traditions while making new developments. In this atmosphere, the skills of athletes improved so quickly that in the two and a half years from 1979, they set a pace unprecedented in Chinese sports: they broke 25 world records, won 22 world titles and took 598 gold medals in international competitions, 326 in 1980 alone. In the first half of 1981, the Chinese men's volleyball team rebounded from a two-game deficit to take the last three games to defeat the south Korean team and join the Chinese women's team in victory at the Asian Zone World Cup Preliminaries — both qualifying to compete in the World Cup volleyball tournaments. In the 36th World Table Tennis Championships held in 1981, Chinese players put on a show of force unprecedented in 55 years of world table tennis championships by winning all the seven titles and taking the runner-up position in all the five individual events. They thus maintained the leading position China has held for 20 years in world table tennis. These brilliant athletic successes not only bring credit to the men and women who achieved them but have bolstered the spirit of the entire Chinese nation, particularly the young people who seek to emulate the hard work embodied in athletic achievement to build up their country. Among those making valuable contributions to the progress of sports in New China have been sports men and women from China's various nationalities, compatriots in Taiwan, Hongkong and Macao, and Chinese residents overseas.

In the past 30 years or more, Chinese athletes have had friendly contacts — some 4,000 involving an estimated 60,000 people — with over 120 other countries and regions. More than 150 Chinese instructors of 14 sports, including table tennis, badminton, volleyball, basketball and gymnastics, are currently working in 34 countries. These contacts have strengthened the friendship between the Chinese people and the people of other countries in the world and promoted sports at home which are avidly followed through news and television coverage.

Among China's sports publications are the magazine *New Sports*, the newspaper *Sports News*, and the English-edition magazine, *Chinese Sports*. The People's Physical Culture Publishing House has brought out some 168 million copies of books dedicated to sports since its founding.

Following the International Olympic Committee's restoration of China's legitimate rights in November 1979, China by the first half of 1981 had become a member country in 40 international sports organizations. Having entered the international arena, Chinese athletes are determined to intensify their training and improve their skills to compete with the best teams and strongest rivals in the world on a wider scale and at a higher level, "to excel in Asia and compete with the world".

At the same time, all those involved in sports in China — both officials and participants — can clearly see that New China must also work hard to close what is still a considerable gap between China and other countries in sports standards and education. New China still lags far behind in skills and levels in many individual sports. Looking forward, in the 1980s, Chinese sports workers will exert their utmost efforts to raise the general health standard of the nation, better the skills and levels of the various sports and contribute to China's socialist cultural development. Plans include making new progress in the sports activities of all people while concentrating on first developing public sports in the cities. More scientific training will produce an even stronger contingent of athletes who will be better equipped to achieve good scores in the Olympic Games, Asian Games and other major international competitions. Contacts with international sports organizations will be strengthened, and exchange in sports with other countries actively conducted so as to promote understanding and friendship between the Chinese people and peoples of other countries and to improve sports skills. Finally, sports activities will be conducted as part of the cultural development programme, as part of the effort to inspire the people with high public moral principles, give vigour to the national spirit and enrich the people's cultural life.

National Games Held in the People's Republic of China

National Games	*First*	*Second*	*Third*	*Fourth*
Time	Sept. 13-Oct. 3, 1959	Sept. 11-28, 1965	Sept. 12-28, 1975	Sept. 15-30, 1979
Place	Beijing	Beijing	Beijing	Beijing
No. of sports events	36	22	Adult 28 Junior 8	Adult 34 Junior 2
No. of group performances	6	1	6	1
No. of athletes participating	10,658	5,922	12,497	15,189
World records broken	4 records by 7 persons on 4 occasions	9 records by 24 persons on 10 occasions	3 records by 1 team and 4 persons on 6 occasions	8 records by 7 persons on 8 occasions (including 3 junior world records by 2 persons on 3 occasions)

World records equalled	—	—	2 records by 2 persons on 2 occasions	3 records by 3 persons on 3 occasions
National records broken	106 records by 664 persons on 884 occasions	130 records by 330 persons on 469 occasions	62 records by 49 teams and 83 persons on 197 occasions	102 records by 36 teams and 204 persons on 376 occasions
National junior records broken	—	—	58 records by 4 teams and 36 persons on 144 occasions	5 records by 2 teams and 6 persons on 10 occasions
Name of group callisthenics	*Nationwide Celebrations*	*Paean to the Revolution*	*Song of the Red Flag*	*The New Long March*
No. of people participating in group callisthenics	8,000	16,000	23,000	16,000

Note: The group performance at the Fourth National Games was the large-scale callisthenics *The New Long March.*

SUCCESSES WON BY CHINESE ATHLETES IN 1980

As China resumed and developed its relations with more international sports organizations in 1980, the first year after China was restored to its legitimate rights on the International Olympic Committee, Chinese athletes made more extensive international contacts. They participated for the first time in the Winter Olympic Games and in a number of other high-level international tournaments where they competed with the world's top teams and best athletes. The Chinese athletes, however, boycotted the Moscow Summer Olympic Games on account of the Soviet invasion of Afghanistan.

In 1980, Chinese sports men and women won many medals in international competitions. Among their honours were: 3 world titles in Table Tennis and Gymnastics World Cups; 22 junior titles in world college and secondary school students' competitions; 19 runners-up and 21 third places in 11 world tournaments; 290-plus first places in more than 60 Asian and other multi-national competitions. In national and international tournaments, Chinese athletes broke or surpassed 7 world records and equalled 3, and bettered a number of Asian records and many national records.

Chinese table tennis players continued to hold their leading position in the world, winning all the team titles in the 11 major international matches in which they participated. Chinese gymnastics, diving and men's and women's volleyball teams, which have been reinforced by newcomers and made fairly rapid progress in recent years, again proved themselves to be among the best in the world. In 11 major international competitions, Chinese gymnasts won 51 championship titles. The Chinese sports acrobatics team and women's chess team took part in international matches for the first time in 1980 and won notable successes. In military sports,

Chinese athletes broke or surpassed a number of world records in parachute jumping, aeroplane modelling and shooting in both national and international competitions.

Good results were achieved also in weightlifting and archery. Track and field and swimming, which had made little headway for more than 10 years, also began to pick up.

In 1980, Chinese athletes also obtained some successes and improved their skills in different degrees in competitions in badminton, men's basketball, tennis, hockey, handball, baseball, softball, ice hockey, speed skating, water polo, canoeing, boat race, *xiangqi* (Chinese chess) and *weiqi* (go).

World Championships Won by Chinese Athletes in 1980

Event	*Winner*	*Tournament*	*Date*	*Place*
Men's singles	Guo Yaohua	First Table Tennis World Cup	Aug. 31	Hongkong
Men's parallel bars	Li Yuejiu	Gymnastics World Cup	Oct. 26	Toronto, Canada
Men's rings	Huang Yubin	Gymnastics World Cup	Oct. 26	Toronto, Canada

World Records Broken or Surpassed by Chinese Athletes in 1980

Event		*Result*	*Winner*	*Tournament*	*Date*	*Place*
Weightlifting	52 kg-class snatch	112 kg	Wu Shude (Guangxi)	National Weightlifting Championships	Apr. 5	Nanning
Shooting	Running bore (mixed run)	390 pts.	Yu Jiping (Shaanxi)	Sino-American Friendship Contest	Sept. 4	Beijing
Model aeroplanes	F3A-53	139.80 km/hr	Zhu Chuangao (Inner Mongolia)	National Aeromodel Contest	Sept. 15	Taiyuan
〃	FIB-4	156.79 km/hr	Sun Yi (Heilongjiang)	〃	Oct. 19	Chengdu
Parachuting	4-man team work	Formation 16	Chinese team	China-Canada-U.S. Friendship Contest	Nov. 26	Guangzhou

Model ships	A3	12"02 (149.750 km/hr)	Ge Meng (Zhejiang)	National Model Ship Contest	Oct. 5	Guangzhou
"	"	12"75 (141.176 km/hr)	Zhang Jianguo (Guangdong)	"	"	"
"	"	13"77 (130.719 km/hr)	Wang Junru (Shanghai)	"	"	"
"	"	14"04 (128.205 km/hr)	Wang Feng (Guizhou)	"	"	"
"	"	10"97 (164.084 km/hr)	Ge Meng (Zhejiang)	"	Oct. 7	"
"	"	13"76 (130.814 km/hr)	Wang Jianzhong (Fujian)	"	"	"
"	"	14"44 (124.654 km/hr)	Han Yongjin (Henan)	"	"	"

"	"	13"20 (136.364 km/hr)	Zhao Mingwu (Hunan)	"	Oct. 8	"
"	"	14"82 (121.457 km/hr)	Deng Qiansheng (Jiangxi)	"	"	"
"	A2	12"85 140.078 km/hr)	Su Weibin (Guangdong)	"	"	"

World Records Equalled by Chinese Athletes in 1980

Event		*Result*	*Winner*	*Tournament*	*Date*	*Place*
Shooting	Women's smallbore rifle: 60 shots prone	598 pts.	Sun Xiuping (Qinghai)	National Shooting Contest	Sept. 8	Zhengzhou
Parachuting	4-man team work	Formation 13	August 1st Team	National Parachuting Contest	Nov. 6	Guangzhou
"	8-man team work	Formation 10	"	China-Canada-U.S. Friendship Contest	Nov. 27	"

National Records Broken in 1980

	No. of Events		No. of Athletes (No. of Teams in Brackets)		No. of Times Records Broken	
	Total	Women's	Total	Women	Total	Women
Track & field	17	6	26 (2)	8	42	13
Swimming	26	13	24 (5)	11 (4)	116	51
Weightlifting	14		18		35	
Speed skating	5	4	7	5	12	10
Archery	16	5	7 (12)	3 (2)	43	6
Shooting	7	3	8 (2)	2 (1)	10	3
Parachuting	2	1	(9)	(4)	11	5

Gliding	3	1	6	2	5	2
Model aeroplanes	4		9		9	
Motorboating	7	4	14	8	28	16
Model ships	5		9		10	
Underwater swimming	14	7	43 (9)	18 (6)	145	58
Total	120	44	171 (39)	57 (17)	466	164

National Junior Records Broken in 1980

	No. of Events		*No. of Athletes (No. of Teams in Brackets)*		*No. of Times Records Broken*	
	Total	Girls'	Total	Girls	Total	Girls
Track & field	19	7	26 (1)	11 (1)	40	21
Swimming	15	8	14	9	53	27
Weightlifting	11		10		23	
Speed skating	1	1	1	1	1	1
Total	46	16	51 (1)	21 (1)	117	49

SUCCESSES ACHIEVED BY CHINESE ATHLETES IN 1981

Chinese athletes reaped the greatest number of successes ever in 1981, winning 25 world titles in 9 sports and carrying home 295 gold medals for 22 events in international competitions in which more than three countries participated. Eight world records were broken or surpassed by 10 Chinese athletes on 11 occasions, and 3 world records were equalled by 2 Chinese athletes and 1 Chinese team. In competitions held in China and abroad, Chinese athletes also created 124 new national records, some measuring up to world levels and many surpassing Asian records.

In the 17 years between 1949 and 1965, Chinese athletes won a total of only 13 championship titles. In 1980 they won 3. In 1981, they competed in a great number of world championships and World Cup competitions to secure more titles than any other year. In these generally recognized top-level competitions, Chinese athletes scored remarkable successes in table tennis, women's volleyball, gymnastics, sports acrobatics, model ships, shooting, chess, badminton, diving, archery and weightlifting. Their internationally acclaimed victories in table tennis and women's volleyball were of great significance in the history of Chinese sports. Chinese players carried off all seven championship titles at the 36th World Table Tennis Championships and were runners-up in all the individual events — a truly remarkable accomplishment that had never before happened in the 55 years of world table tennis championships. When the Chinese women's volleyball team emerged victorious at the Third World Cup — winning all the seven games it played — it made a breakthrough in that a Chinese team for the first time won a championship title in one of the three major ball games — basketball, volleyball and football.

The splendid victories scored by Chinese athletes in 1981 have inspired the people of the whole country with patriotic determination to work hard for the renewed prosperity and strength of China. People of all walks of life now speak about the "pingpong spirit" and the "women volleyballers' spirit" as they undertake their own efforts to win distinctions for the country. This has given rise to a "sports fever" and "patriotic fever" which have become a powerful impetus to the development of sports in China. Chinese athletes are at present undergoing intensive training in preparation for winning even greater honours at the coming 1982 Asian Games, the National Games of 1983 and the Olympic Games scheduled for 1984.

World Championships Won by Chinese Athletes in 1981

Event	*Winner(s)*	*Tournament*	*Date*	*Place*
Weiqi (go)	Shao Zhenzhong	Third World Amateur Go Championships	Mar. 10-14	Tokyo, Japan
Men's team event	Chinese men's team	36th World Table Tennis Championships	Apr. 13-26	Yugoslavia
Women's team event	Chinese women's team	"	"	"
Men's singles	Guo Yaohua	"	"	"
Women's singles	Tong Ling	"	"	"
Men's doubles	Li Zhenshi & Cai Zhenhua	"	"	"
Women's doubles	Zhang Deying & Cao Yanhua	"	"	"

Mixed doubles	Xie Saike & Huang Junqun	″	″	″
Women's spring-board	Shi Meiqin	Second World Cup Diving Tournament	June 12-14	Mexico
Men's platform	Li Hongping	″	″	″
Women's platform	Chen Xiaoxia	″	″	″
Men's singles	Chen Changjie	First World Games Badminton Tournament	July 28	U.S.A.
Men's doubles	Sun Zhi'an & Yao Ximing	″	″	″
Women's singles	Zhang Ailing	″	″	″
Women's doubles	Zhang Ailing & Liu Xia	″	″	″
F2B	Wei Yuming	Second World Championships in Model Ships	Aug. 19-23	GDR

Women's trio all-round	Feng Yanfang, Cai Yu & Liu Yingmei	Third World Cup Sports Acrobatics	Sept. 4-6	Widnau, Switzerland
Men's four all-round	Lin Yuanxiang, He Jidong, Chen Tie & Liang Jiankun	"	"	"
Women's pair individual (set 2)	Zeng Jianhua & Yin Wu	"	"	"
Men's four individual (set 1)	Lin Yuanxiang, He Jidong, Chen Tie & Liang Jiankun	"	"	"
Women's team skeet	Wu Lanying, Feng Meimei & Shao Weiping	42nd World Clay-Pigeon Shooting Championships	Oct. 26	Tucuman, Argentina
Women's individual skeet	Wu Lanying	"	Oct. 27	"

Women's volleyball	Women's volleyball team	Third World Cup Volleyball Tournament	Nov. 7-16	Japan
Pommel horse	Li Xiaoping	21st World Gymnastics Championships	Nov. 23-29	USSR
Men's floor exercise	Li Yuejiu	"	"	"

Chinese Athletes Won 295 Titles in International Competitions in 1981

Event	*No. of Titles Won*	*Event*	*No, of Titles Won*
Basketball	5	Diving	9
Volleyball	8	Canoeing	5
Football	2	Rowing	7
Handball	1	Shooting	4
Table tennis	70	Archery	4
Badminton	10	Parachuting	9
Tennis	11	Chess	6
Track & field	36	Judo	1
Weightlifting	28	Fencing	3
Gymnastics	66	Aeromodel	1
Swimming	8	Water polo	1

World Records Broken or Surpassed by Chinese Athletes in 1981

Event		*Record*	*Winner*	*Tournament*	*Date*	*Place*
Weight-lifting	56 kg-class snatch	126.5 kg	Wu Shude	13th Asian Weightlifting Championships	Aug. 16	Nagoya, Japan
Model ships	A2	12″3 (146.341 km/hr)	Hu Sheng-gao	National Model Ship Contest	June 9	Hangzhou
″	″	11″6 (155.172 km/hr)	″	″	June 10	″
″	″	11″9 (151.260 km/hr)	Guo Shankuang	″	″	″
″	″	13″3 (135.338 km/hr)	Gao Baokang	″	″	″
″	″	11″4 (157.895 km/hr)	Hu Sheng-gao	Second World Championships in Model Ships	Aug. 19-23	GDR

″	A3	13″ (138.461 km/hr)	Han Yongjin	National Model Ship Contest	June 9	Hangzhou
″	″	11″2 (160.714 km/hr)	Ge Meng	″	June 10	″
″	″	11″5 (156.522 km/hr)	Wang Feng	″	June 11	″
″	″	12″1 (148.760 km/hr)	Wang Junru	″	June 12	″
″	″	13″5 (133.333 km/hr)	Yu Lei	″	″	″
″	″	11″01 (163.488 km/hr)	Ge Meng	Second World Championships in Model Ships	Aug. 19-23	GDR
″	B1	8″7 (206.896 km/hr)	Chen Liang	National Model Ship Contest	June 12	Hangzhou

Shooting	Running boar (mixed run)	390 pts.	Xie Yili	National Elite Meet	Apr. 23	Changsha
"	Women's skeet	194 pts.	Wu Lanying	National Shooting Tournament	Sept. 20	Shijia-zhuang
"	"	194 pts.	Feng Meimei	"	"	"
"	Men's air pistol	395 pts.	Liu Zhenghong	"	Oct. 26	Hangzhou
"	Centre-fire small-bore pistol	593 pts.	Yan Cuiqing	"	Oct. 27	"

World Records Equalled by Chinese Athletes in 1981

Event	*Result*	*Winner(s)*	*Tournament*	*Date*	*Place*
Running boar (mixed run) (team event)	1,533 pts.	Yu Jiping, Chu Gang, Wang Zhong-yuan & Xie Yili	1981 World Running Boar Shooting Championships	Oct. 16-21	Argentina
Running boar (mixed run) (individual event)	387 pts.	Yu Jiping	"	"	"
Women's centre-fire small-bore pistol	592 pts.	Wen Zhifang	National Elite Meet	Apr. 22	Changsha

National Records Broken in 1981

	No. of Events		*No. of Athletes (No. of Teams in Brackets)*		*No. of Times Records Broken*	
	Total	Women's	Total	Women	Total	Women
Total	124	43	135 (43)	46 (18)	395	125
Track & field	20	5	20 (3)	4 (1)	45	10
Swimming	20	9	19 (19)	10 (7)	65	28
Weightlifting	14		14		41	
Speed skating	12	6	12	5	33	17
Track cycling	3	3	4 (1)	4 (1)	6	6
Archery	18	7	7 (2)	2 (1)	42	9

Shooting	10	3	8 (6)	4 (2)	17	9
Parachuting	5	3	2 (8)	2 (4)	15	11
Gliding	1		2		1	
Model aeroplanes	3		4		4	
Motorboating	2	1	17	9	37	19
Model ships	2		7		18	
Underwater swimming	14	6	19 (4)	6 (2)	71	16

National Junior Records Broken in 1981

	No. of Events		*No. of Athletes (No. of Teams in Brackets)*		*No. of Times Records Broken*	
	Total	Girls'	Total	Girls	Total	Girls
Total	32	11	27 (1)	9 (1)	66	23
Track & field	12	6	12 (1)	5 (1)	20	12
Swimming	9	5	5	4	19	11
Weightlifting	11		10		27	

2. PUBLIC SPORTS

Playing an important role in China's cultural development, public sports include all sports activities in schools, among workers and employees, peasants, the armed forces, children, the aged, the disabled and the handicapped.

In economically and culturally backward old China, when most people lived in poverty and sports remained the diversions of a tiny minority, there were no public sports to speak of. Only with the tremendous development of sports in post-liberation years has it been possible for the broad masses of people to use sports as an important means to build up their health and enrich their cultural life.

Sports in Schools Because the physical condition of China's 200 million young people and children studying in schools and colleges has a vital bearing on their completing their studies and participating in the construction of their country, the work of public sports is focused on sports in school when young people are in important stages of bodily growth and are acquiring both knowledge and abilities. The Chinese government has adopted a series of important measures to promote physical culture and sports in schools: Physical education is an integral part of the educational policy in school programmes to assure that students develop in an all-round way — morally, intellectually and physically. A unified teaching programme in physical education has been drawn up, applicable throughout the country. First-year and second-year college students and all secondary and primary school students are required to attend two periods of P. E. classes and to participate in extracurricular sports activities at least twice each week. In addition, students are expected to take part in morning exercises, exercises during the breaks between classes and eye exercises. Physical education institutes have been established while physical education departments have been set up in some colleges and universities.

In 1979, all the schools and colleges in the country began to implement experimentally the "Provisional Regulations for Physical Culture in Institutes of Higher Learning" and "Provisional Regulations for Physical Culture in Secondary and Elementary Schools" (Draft) which define the tasks, content, forms of organization, and rules and regulations concerning work in physical education and sports in colleges and schools. For instance, a system of checks on attendance and examinations was instituted by which students who fail to attend more than one-third of the sports classes receive no credit at the end of the term, and those whose grades are below "Good" cannot be elected as students of "Three Good's" (ideologically, academically and physically). Sports also became one of the subjects which determines whether a student will be promoted to the next grade. The Ministry of Education stipulated in 1981 that college and university applicants who have passed the "National Standards of Physical Fitness" tests will be given priority for admission when their other qualifications are the same as those applicants who have not passed, and that it will gradually become universal practice that all senior secondary school graduates must, in general, pass the "National Standards of Physical Fitness" tests before they can apply for admission at colleges and universities. These stipulations move towards correcting any tendency to neglect physical training.

To cultivate talent and cater to students' love for and interest in sports, sports teams are organized in all schools and universities. The various provinces, municipalities and autonomous regions have also selected a number of schools and universities to specialize in one or several kinds of sports. According to statistics from 24 provinces, municipalities and autonomous regions, 3,486 secondary and primary schools and seven universities have been thus selected. More schools have been selected by authorities at the prefectural and county levels. These schools and their sports teams — veritable cradles of sports talent — provide two or three periods of special training a week, each lasting 90 minutes. More than 14,000 students in 123 schools selected by Shanghai municipality and 301 schools by Shanghai municipal districts are receiving such special training in sports guided by 911 physical training teachers who serve as coaches. The northeastern city of Dalian is noted for football, a popular sport, in more than 490 out of the city's 500-plus secondary and primary schools. Today, one in every five players on the nation's 16 Class-A football teams is from Dalian. In the past 30-plus years, nearly 1,000 of the city's football players have played on the national, provincial and city teams. The No. 18 Secondary School in Qingdao specializes in field and track sports. Three high jumpers from that school have cleared 2.00 metres. Since 1970, three of its students have broken three national junior records, 27 have bettered 11 provincial junior records on 91 occasions; 20 of its students have been enrolled in the city's spare-time sports schools and 24 recruited by the provincial, city or national teams.

Pre-school children also participate in sports. Exercises and outdoor games are popular among children in kindergartens. Some cities have sponsored children's sports meetings and athletic exhibitions. Most parks and other public places are equipped with children's recreational grounds. All this has provided favourable conditions for the healthy growth of the younger generation.

National Standards of Physical Fitness These were put into practice throughout the country after approval by the State Council in 1974 to provide basic requirements of physical fitness for young people and children. The government first promulgated the "System of Physical Training for Labour and National Defence" in 1954 which was renamed "Standards of Physical Fitness for Young People" in 1964, and "National Standards of Physical Fitness" in 1974. The standards are different for different sexes and age groups. There are now four age groups: Children: 10-12 years old; Junior 1: 13-15 years old; Junior 2: 16-17 years old; and Youth: 18-30 years old. Those who have passed the tests are given a badge and a certificate.

The setting up of standards of physical fitness has encouraged young people and children to take part consciously and actively in physical training and has helped to build up courage, willpower and a collective spirit. In the 20 and more years before 1980, some 80.6 million people have met the standards of fitness of different classes. In 1981, specialists were called together to revise the standards in the light of the experience gained in the previous years.

Sports for Workers and Employees Trade unions at different levels regard it as an important task to conduct sports activities among workers and employees, the main force in China's socialist construction. Various sports activities in factories, mines and other enterprises are carried out under the principle that they be voluntarily pursued in leisure hours, on small scale and rich in variety.

The All-China Federation of Trade Unions sponsored the First National Workers' Games in October 1955, for some 1,700 worker-athletes. Eight national records were broken by 11 athletes in track and field events, weight-lifting and bicycle race. In 1957, 74 basketball, volleyball and football teams composed of workers and employees, eight of which were national Class-A teams, took part in the national league matches. In the 1950s, the ranks of workers and employees produced 20 Masters of Sports, 62 First-Class Sportsmen and a large number of Second- and Third-Class Sportsmen. Famous table tennis players like Xu Yinsheng, Wang Chuanyao, Sun Meiying, Zhang Xielin and Zhuang Jiafu were all workers and employees. Many model workers and advanced individuals — those workers who have excelled in production — have been pace-setters in the sports as well.

Today, workers and employees are actively engaged in all kinds of sports. More than 1.2 million railway workers and employees who belong to the Locomotive Sports Association regularly do limbering-up exercises to radio music, and 570,000 take part in winter physical training. About a third of all the workers and employees in the city of Tangshan and in the Anshan Iron and Steel Company of northeast China regularly participate in sports. Trade unions at various levels are also keen organizers of sports competitions.

Limbering-Up Exercises Done to Broadcast Music More people participate in these sets of exercises for stretching and strengthening the limbs and trunk, done to music broadcast by radio stations, than in any other sport. The exercises are simple to do in all seasons and do not require special grounds or facilities. Since 1951, the State Physical Culture and Sports Commission has successively promulgated six sets of exercises for adults, four sets for teenagers, and five sets for children. The government stipulates that factories, mines, other enterprises, offices and schools offer two 10-minute breaks, one in the morning and another in the afternoon, for physical exercises, and the music for doing limbering-up exercises is broadcast by the central and local radio stations during these breaks. Special exercises have been designed for iron and steel workers, coal miners and textile workers. School students also do eye exercises.

Peasants' Sports Sports activities at the village or production brigade and team level — practised in the early morning or in the evening — combine a great variety of local sports with militia training and festival celebrations. Some better-off communes, production brigades and teams have paid constant attention to developing sports activities. The Beiling Commune in Hai'an County, Jiangsu Province, for example, holds all-commune peasant games on May Day every year, the 1981 games being its 17th. Events include racing, long jump, grenade-throwing, cycling, tug-of-war, basketball, table tennis, physical exercises and such characteristic village sports as bayonet exercises by militiamen and a *taijiquan* (shadow boxing) demonstration by older people.

In the past year, as rural economic conditions have taken a turn for the better, village cultural centres have begun to appear in the countryside, which include sports in their activities, encouraging the development of athletics in rural areas. According to statistics from 12 provinces, including Guangdong and Shandong, more than

1,100 villages and townships have established such cultural centres.

"Homes of Sports" Over the years, as public sports have become increasingly popular, "homes of sports" have emerged across the length and breadth of the country. These are areas which, according to local interests and customs, have developed one or two kinds of sports as their specialities. With long practice, they continuously consolidate and improve their standards for these sports to turn them into their traditions. These "homes of sports" provide centres for popularizing and improving sports and point to the direction in which China's public sports should develop. Many top athletes in China have come from these "homes of sports".

China's "home of swimmers" is Dongguan County in Guangdong Province where — with its many rivers and lakes — at least 50 per cent of the population can be considered swimmers. Swimming is so popular in the county's Daojiao People's Commune that of a population of 40,000, some 30,000 are swimmers. More than 25,000 students in the county participate on their school swimming teams or study in their schools' sports classes, not to mention the 1,000-plus who are receiving systematic training in 11 spare-time sports schools. Some 246 swimmers from the county have at one time or another swum on national teams.

Other provinces and cities where swimming is popular include Jiangsu Province where over four million people took part in river-crossing swims in 1977, Hubei Province where over 4.7 million are swimming fans, and the city of Nanning in the Guangxi Zhuang Autonomous Region where some 10,000 people participated in a winter swim in the Yongjiang River over a distance of 16 kilometres.

China's "home of weightlifting" is Stone Dragon Town, Dongguan County, Guangdong Province, a small rural township with a small population, which yet has produced several dozen people who have won the title of Master of Sports. Of the 31 world weightlifting records set by Chinese athletes since the founding of the People's Republic, 16 have been by weightlifters from Stone Dragon. Well-known weightlifters from Stone Dragon include Chen Jingkai, Chen Manlin, Ye Haobo, Li Jiyuan, Liu Hangyuan and Chen Weiqiang as well as budding young weightlifters like Ye Ganbo, Ye Lianfa and Ye Haotang. There are many families of weightlifters in the township. Chen Jingkai and Chen Manlin are Chen Weiqiang's uncles, and all three are world record setters. Chen Zhi, who has been engaged in weightlifting for over 20 years and won the national title of Distinguished Weightlifting Instructor of Spare-Time Sports School, is Chen Jingkai's elder brother. Weightlifting is practised in all of the town's nine primary schools, and a township weightlifting contest among primary school pupils is held every year. This method of training weightlifters from childhood has proved very effective. Some instructors say that weightlifters from Stone Dragon, with their good basic training, start at a higher level and progress more quickly than most. They are able to get good results after a short period of intensive training.

China's "home of volleyball" is Taishan County in Guangdong Province. According to statistics made available in 1972, there were 2,100 volleyball courts and 5,300 volleyball teams in the county, which was almost one for every production team of the people's communes.

Over 300 top players from the county have played on national, provincial and city teams.

Gaixian County in Liaoning Province and Zhangzhou in Fujian Province are also well-known centres for volleyball. Joining them in recent years are Zizhou in Shaanxi Province, Kaiping and Wenchang in Guangdong Province and Yanbian in Jilin Province.

China's "home of football" is Meixian County in Guangdong Province where almost each of the 30 local communes as well as the local secondary and primary schools has its own football field and team. Children often use a coconut instead of a proper ball in their spirited matches. The Bingcun Commune is best known for its many "football families" and "multi-generation football fans". About 70 per cent of the adults in the commune frequently take pleasure in kicking the ball. The commune boasts of an effective three-level football training network covering secondary schools, primary schools and kindergartens. Even the kindergartens have their baby football teams. Since the first special sports schools were set up in Meixian, they have trained more than 2,000 football players, 120 of whom have been chosen to represent the country or province, becoming key players in their teams.

Lüda in Liaoning Province and Yanbian in Jilin Province are also traditional football centres. Santai in Sichuan Province, Jinxian in Liaoning Province, Lijiang in Yunnan Province and Wuhua in Guangdong Province have recently gone in for football as their main sport which is steadily gaining popularity.

China's "home of track and field athletes" is Putian County in Fujian Province, followed in recent years by Huaide County in Jilin Province. Yexian in Shandong

Province specializes in medium- and long-distance running. All the schools there have running teams. A number of the county's runners have represented China in international competitions. Song Meihua, champion in the women's 1,500-metre race at the Seventh Asian Games, received her early basic training in Yexian.

Winter in China's northernmost province of Heilongjiang is very cold, but ideal for sports on ice and snow. Its Harbin is known as the "City of Ice", for at the end of 1980 its artificial skating rinks covered a total area of 480,000 square metres and were frequented by 230,000 regular skaters. The counties under the jurisdiction of the prefecture of Songhuajiang where there are a total of 149 skiing courses are known as the "home of skiing".

Wushu, or martial arts, have been a favourite sport of the people of Cangzhou in Hebei Province since ancient times. It has thus become known as the "home of *wushu*". At the National Traditional *Wushu* Meet held in Taiyuan in May 1980, five of the eight members of the Hebei team were from Cangzhou, and three of the four gold medals won by the team were thanks to Cangzhou athletes.

Other "homes of sports" include Dongan County in Hunan Province, of *wushu*; the Inner Mongolia Autonomous Region, and Xinxian County in Shanxi Province, of wrestling; Wuqiao County in Hebei Province and Xinzhou County in Hubei Province, of gymnastics.

Sports for the Aged China has 47 million people who are 65 or older. In September 1979, the All-China Sports Federation passed a resolution for the establishment of an association of sports for the aged. A preparatory meeting was held in Beijing in May 1981 and the association will be formerly established in 1982. Local associations of sports or a single sport for the aged have already been set up in Beijing, Shanghai, Changchun and among railway workers. Similar sports and physical training organizations have come into existence in other provinces and municipalities, too. The five district associations of sports for the aged in Shanghai have increased their membership to 2,500 who take part in contests, attend lectures, take regular physical check-ups and go out on athletic tours. Such activities have been well received by China's senior citizens.

For many years, a considerable number of older people in China's cities and towns have been doing regular morning exercises. Coaching centres for *taijiquan* (shadow boxing), *qigong* (breathing exercises) and *liangong shibafa* (18 exercises of martial arts) have sprung up one after another. Over 100,000 older people in Shanghai alone and about 40,000 in Beijing take part in these activities. Elderly citizens in Shanghai and other places have organized their own football, basketball, tennis and long-distance running teams. At the time of the Fourth National Games held in September 1979, 60 aged men and women runners from Beijing's old people's long-distance running team held an exhibition race.

At the National Workers' and Employees' Long-Distance Race by Correspondence held in 1979, a special race was held for elderly runners. At a long-distance race for the elderly and middle-aged held in Hangzhou, the oldest among the men runners was 88 years old and among the women runners, 71 years old. There is always a race for the elderly in the New Year and Spring Festival cross-country and round-the-city races held every year in Beijing, Chengdu, Changzhou and other places. Some 160 men and women members of the old people's New Long

March Long-Distance Running Team in Xi'an held a symbolic race to cover the distance from Xi'an to Beijing.

In February and November 1979, the old people's long-distance running organizations in Beijing, Shanghai, Chengdu and Kunming twice received the friendly visiting delegation of the Japanese "Sea Turtle" Long-Distance Association for the Aged and Middle-Aged headed by Hideo Okada. Races and discussions were held between Japanese and Chinese runners.

In May 1981, more than 300 old and middle-aged long-distance runners from six cities (including Shanghai, Hangzhou and Wuxi) travelled to Wuxi for long-distance races and a sight-seeing tour by boat on Taihu Lake. This self-financed and warmly enjoyed occasion was initiated and organized by the Health Building and Long-Distance Running Association and other people's sports organizations of Wuxi. They have decided that in the future the six cities will take turns organizing the event.

Sports for the Disabled Sports help disabled persons to overcome their disabilities and enhance their health in body and spirit by awakening their love for life and inspiring their morale. As part of its general concern for the life and education of the disabled, the people's government gives special attention to their sports activities. Schools for the deaf-mute and the blind, like ordinary schools, have two periods of sports classes every week as well as twice a week extracurricular sports activities. Sports activities in welfare factories for the disabled are organized by the trade unions there. In the sanatoria for the disabled and rest homes for disabled soldiers, sports are an important means for restoring health.

There are as yet no sports organizations for the disabled in China. Their sports are under the jurisdiction of the China Association of Deaf-Mutes and the China Welfare Association of the Blind, assisted by the State Physical Culture and Sports Commission, the Ministry of Education, the Ministry of Civil Affairs and the All-China Federation of Trade Unions.

A national track and field and swimming contest, which was sponsored by the China Association of Deaf-Mutes and in which 60 athletes from 16 provinces and cities participated, was held in Beijing in 1957. A basketball tournament for deaf-mutes held in 1959 was participated in by teams from every province and municipality in China. Several national sports meets of the blind, some played off through correspondence, have been held in China following the first National Sports Meet of the Young Blind held in Shanghai in June 1957 under the sponsorship of the China Welfare Association of the Blind, the State Physical Culture and Sports Commission and the Ministry of Education. Sports meetings of the deaf-mute and the blind have also been held in some other municipalities and provinces. A track and field meet was held in 1980 between schools for blind children in Beijing, Tianjin, Tangshan and Zhangjiakou. In early 1981, blind persons in Shanghai competed in a Chinese chess tournament, and Huangshi in Hubei Province witnessed a track and field meet of deaf-mutes from eight organizations in the city. An athletic meet of the blind and the deaf-mute sponsored by the municipality of Beijing lasted from April 15 to the end of May 1981, participated in by 740 sportsmen from 68 organizations.

In 1981, designated by the United Nations as the International Year of disabled persons, China set up an organizing committee for this purpose. Composed of responsible members from more than 20 departments including the State Bureau of Labour, the Ministry of Civil Affairs and the State Physical Culture and Sports Commission, the committee organized the activities — including sports — related to the International Year.

Jogging Many consider jogging, which requires no special equipment or place to practise, the perfect sport. It is steadily developing into a popular sport in China today. Between November 1979 and March 1980, 6.58 million students, workers and employees in Liaoning Province alone regularly took part in long-distance running. Many of its schools and other basic units organized a symbolic Liaoning-Beijing long-distance running in which runners, without leaving their cities or towns, covered the distance between Liaoning and Beijing. There was a mass upsurge in winter physical training in the city of Xi'an under the slogan, "Run 200 kilometres in 100 winter days." The long-distance run organized in the city on New Year's Day 1980 was joined by 15,000 people.

Public round-the-city or cross-country races on New Year's Day or during the Spring Festival have become a tradition in many cities. Such races were held on New Year's Day 1981 in Shanghai, Wuhan, Lanzhou, Hohhot, Nanning, Hefei, Shijiazhuang, Xi'an, Chengdu and other cities, while the tradition in Beijing, Chongqing and some other cities is to hold round-the-city races during the Spring Festival.

Therapeutic Exercises Exercises, such as *taijiquan* (shadow boxing), *qigong* (breathing exercises) and *wuqinxi* (five-animal exercises) have become a chief aid in curing many chronic diseases in many of China's sanatoria which have set up their own departments of therapeutic exercises. In the seven years since its founding, the Guangzhou No. 12 People's Hospital has combined exercise therapy with medicine to treat 2,338 patients suffering from various kinds of chronic diseases. Some 285 were completely cured while the condition of 1,867 improved. The efficacy rate was 92 per cent, one-third higher than that with medicine alone. The Taihu Lake Workers' Sanatorium has succeeded in curing many sufferers of chronic diseases through therapeutic exercises.

Taijiquan, qigong and *wuqinxi*, which were created by the Chinese people in the course of years of practice, are traditional exercises with a long history. In recent years, therapeutic exercises have become very popular in many cities and towns. Among the best known are *qigong* in Beijing and *liangong shibafa* (18 exercises of martial arts) in Shanghai.

The *Qigong* Research Society set up in Beijing in December 1979 runs 33 *qigong* therapy coaching centres in the city proper. Since that time some 4,044 persons have enrolled in classes lasting three months. Of the 3,159 invalids who take regular *qigong* exercises, 786 have been restored to full health, 1,396 have achieved remarkable improvement, and 696 have made visible improvement. The exercises failed to have any noticeable effect on only 281 persons. *Qigong* exercises at the Tiantan *qigong* centre produced remarkable results in the case of Sun Yanqin, a cancer patient, and Hou Yunxiu, who suffered from heart trouble. Both have now gone back to work.

Liangong shibafa was designed by two doctors from the Dongchang Road Hospital in Shanghai. These exercises have proved effective in curing more than 98 per cent of pains in the neck, shoulder, back and leg as well as cardiac and vascular conditions. Applied in 183 cases in the departments of internal medicine, surgery, traumatology and osteology, the efficacy rate was 95.7 per cent. The Taihu Lake Workers' Sanatorium in Wuxi has achieved 90.6 per cent of cure in treating gastroptosis (a collapse of the stomach into the lower abdomen).

3. NATIONAL TRADITIONAL SPORTS

As part of the valuable cultural legacy of the Chinese nation, traditional sports have been successfully carried forward and developed. This is particularly true of a number of the more popular items.

Wushu *Wushu*, or martial arts, practised for several thousand years by the working people in China for physical training and self-defence, is still immensely popular in both the urban and rural areas today. Chinese *wushu* also has aroused interest among foreigners and is taught in many countries throughout the world.

Wushu is practised in various types of set exercises, either barehanded or with weapons, based on movements employed in fighting, such as kicking, striking, throwing, catching, repelling and stabbing. Performers follow the laws of change from one to the other of two contradictory aspects: attack and defence, advance and retreat, action and inaction, acceleration and deceleration, strength and grace, false move and real move. A unique Chinese national sport, *wushu* builds strong bodies, steels the willpower and gives training in fighting skills.

There are several dozen types of barehanded *wushu* exercises, which include *changquan, nanquan* (southern boxing), *taijiquan* (shadow boxing), and *xingyiquan* (imitation boxing). *Changquan* is subdivided into many schools, including *zhaquan* (Zha's boxing), *huaquan* (Hua's boxing) and *shaolinquan* (Shaolin boxing). *Nanquan* is the collective name of many schools of boxing widely practised in the southern part of China, which are generally based on the movements of the dragon, tiger, leopard, snake and crane. The weapons used in *wushu* exercises are broad sword, spear, double-edged sword, club, nine-sectioned chain and plummet and line, to mention but a few. Weapons are used in practice through several sets of exercises. There are also exercises in pairs, armed or unarmed; with weapon against a bare-handed opponent; and collective exercises. As the sets of *wushu* exercises contain many beautiful, natural body movements, they have become great attractions in Chinese opera where they have been adopted for fighting scenes on stage. Chinese acrobatics have also absorbed the best of the basic *wushu* movements.

Wushu's long history in China includes development by the working people as they engaged in productive labour and struggle. Even in ancient times *wushu* was used in education, physical training and medicine. The famous surgeon Hua Tuo, who lived in the period of the Three Kingdoms (220-280), designed the *wuqinxi* (five-animal exercises) for curing diseases and physical training which has been handed down to the present day. In the course of its development over the centuries, *wushu* has been steadily enriched both in content and form. On the other hand, the ruling class throughout history also introduced feudal superstitious ideas into it, leading it astray or degrading it. This diminished a fine cultural legacy.

After the founding of the People's Republic, *wushu* has undergone sound development. In 1950, the All-China Sports Federation held a symposium on the work of *wushu*. A national exhibition meet of traditional sports took place in 1953, which offered an opportunity for many fine local traditional *wushu* practices which had been hidden in obscurity to be developed and preserved. The guiding principle put forward by the government at the time was to "rediscover, systematize and raise standards". Beginning in 1955, the State Physical Culture and Sports Commission organized groups of *wushu* professionals and sportsmen to rediscover, study and systematize *wushu* sports. *Wushu* books on barehanded exercises and exercises with a sword, spear, club, and other weapons were published. *Wushu* courses are now offered at all physical culture colleges in this country, and *wushu* training classes and coaching centres have been set up in many places. There is also a national *wushu* association. *Wushu* contests were included in all the four National Games held in New China. There have also been many national *wushu* exhibitions and contests, which have helped popularize this branch of China's traditional martial arts. Today, it is a common sight to see groups of *wushu* enthusiasts practising exercises with or without weapon everywhere in the country. "Homes of *wushu*", where there is a long tradition of martial arts, include Dongan County in Hunan Province, Cangzhou County in Hebei Province and Jinan Prefecture in Shandong Province. In Dongan County alone, 40 per cent of the entire population and 70 per cent of the young people take part in *wushu* exercises. The National *Wushu* Demonstration held in the city of Nanning, Guangxi Zhuang Autonomous Region, in May 1979 was unprecedented. A total of 510 exercises were performed. A similar one held in the city of Taiyuan, Shanxi Province, at the end of May 1980 was another grand occasion for rediscovering the almost lost art of *wushu*. It was participated by more than 200 of the best *wushu* masters, who performed 517 exercises, 74 of which won prizes at the meet. The National *Wushu* Demonstration held in Shenyang in May 1981 was even larger and better. Seventy-nine of the 200-plus masters who performed 522 exercises won prizes. Spectators had their eyes opened when some traditional set exercises which had been thought lost were performed by veteran *wushu* masters.

Taijiquan This is a branch of Chinese martial arts with a history of over 300 years. In the 17th century when the rule of the Ming Dynasty was being replaced by that of Qing, wars were frequent. *Wushu* was widely practised by the ordinary people. As a result, a new form of boxing came into being which drew upon and incorporated various other martial arts. In actual fighting, this new form was able to overcome might through supple and clever moves. At the end of the 18th century, a famous master named Wang Zongyue systematized it and named it *taijiquan.* Gaining popularity first in the villages of Henan Province, it spread to Beijing in mid-19th century and later to both urban and rural areas throughout the northern and southern parts of China.

Taijiquan is practised in complete sequences, including barehanded exercises, exercises with an opponent, or with a double-edged sword, broad sword, spear or club. Originally a fighting art, *taijiquan* over the last hundred years — as society developed and its needs became different — gradually became a health-building and therapeutic exercise. It is now a gentle, peaceful art with a minimum of jumps and exertive moves.

In the course of its development, four main schools of *taijiquan* have come into being, the most widely practised being the Yang-style *taijiquan* founded by Yang

Chengfu. This school is characterized by steady, expansive movements. Next comes the Wu-style *taijiquan* founded by Wu Jianquan and known for its closely packed but gentle movements. The Sun-style *taijiquan* of Sun Lutang is noted for its small and agile movements while the Chen-style *taijiquan* of Chen Fake, which retains more of the old traditions, has both powerful and gentle movements.

The millions of people in China who practise *taijiquan* every day usually do it in the early morning in a park, in a playground, in their own courtyards, by a river or along the roadside. Some also do the exercise with a sword. To meet the needs of the masses of devotees, the State Physical Culture and Sports Commission designed a simplified *taijiquan* of 24 typical exercises based on the Yang style, following the principle of eliminating the redundant and keeping the essential while making it easy to learn and practise. This simplified *taijiquan,* also known as the Twenty-Four Exercises, can be practised to the accompaniment of classical national music which proves to be a boon to beginners. Many other newly designed *taijiquan* set exercises for individual and group performances combine the features of various schools. These include *taijiquan* of 48, 66 and 88 exercises, which have greatly enriched the content of this traditional martial art. The People's Physical Culture Publishing House in Beijing has published many books and charts on *taijiquan.* Coaching centres have been set up in many cities, with more than 100 in Beijing alone, where *taijiquan* is taught by several hundred coaches.

Despite their differences in style, the various schools of *taijiquan* are basically the same in essentials and main features. The two most important principles are: 1) Relaxation. It is important to keep the body relaxed and natural and the movements gentle and continuous. Exertion is to be avoided by all means. 2) Serenity. It is important to focus one's attention on the exercise itself and have serenity of mind. *Taijiquan* is an integrated exercise for training the body, the mind and the "vital energy", with the main emphasis on the mind. The mind is to follow the movements of the body. Since *taijiquan* stresses this mental aspect rather than strength, some people call it — not without reason — an exercise of the mind.

It is believed that, with the attention of the practitioners highly concentrated on the physical movements, *taijiquan* can make the cerebral cells recover from overexcitement and functional disorders, which can in turn alter some stubborn physiological patterns and thus help treat such physical disorders as neurasthenia, high blood pressure and ulcers. *Taijiquan* can be practised by both men and women, old and young, the physically strong or weak. It is most suitable for the elderly, sufferers of chronic ailments and those who engage in intellectual work. Since long and persistent practice of *taijiquan* improves one's health, it is regarded as an important therapeutic sport which can prevent and cure illness.

Taijiquan found its way abroad a long time ago and is being practised in many other countries today, particularly in Southeast Asia. The *Taijiquan* Association and *Taijiquan* Liaison Committee in Japan have more than 30 branches across that country. Scores of books on *taijiquan* have been published in the United States since the 1960s. An increasing number of foreign residents in Beijing also have taken an interest in this traditional sport in recent years.

Liangong Shibafa Meaning "eighteen exercises of

martial arts", *liangong shibafa* is a set of new therapeutic exercises which first became popular in Shanghai. According to statistics collected in 1979, more than 100,000 participated in this sport in that city alone. Early in the morning, people can be seen doing this exercise everywhere in the city. *Liangong shibafa,* based on traditional Chinese medicine and *wushu,* also combines knowledge in modern medicine and physical therapy. As a sport, it serves to improve one's health. As a therapeutic method, it is effective in curing a number of ailments, particularly discomforts in the neck, shoulder, back and leg. As the Eighteen Exercises are easy to learn, need no special facilities and can be pursued by the elderly and people who are in frail health, they have been taken up by the broad masses of the people, becoming more and more popular throughout the country.

Qigong Literally meaning "breathing exercises", *qigong* was mentioned in records in China dating as far back as 3,000 years ago. They aim at controlling the mind and regulating the breath to keep fit, live long, overcome disease and strengthen physiological functions.

Health-building *qigong* is a unique Chinese national sport. It is, in fact, both a sport and a kind of physical therapy. There are many schools of health-building *qigong*, but all forms involve three essential aspects: regulation of body position (the exercises are performed in a sitting, lying, standing or walking position), regulation of respiration (including mainly the regulation of breathing and "inner energy"), and regulation of the mind (by directing attention in a certain direction or on a certain spot to attain tranquility and concentration of the mind). The three aspects of the exercises should be coordinated to achieve an equilibrium of the bodily functions to help gain immunity from disease and build a strong constitution. Health-building *qigong* is increasingly popular in China today, especially among older people and patients of chronic diseases.

Therapeutic *qigong* is applied to a patient by a *qigong* practitioner. Since it involves the use of bioelectricity to treat specific diseases, it is a therapeutic method rather than a sport.

Xiangqi *Weiqi* (go), *xiangqi* (Chinese chess) and international chess have been listed in China as national competitive sports, for which national tournaments are held every year. *Weiqi* and *xiangqi* have been known in China from ancient times.

Of the three chess games, *xiangqi* is the most popular throughout the country. It has been estimated that there are about 100 million enthusiasts in China. Chess-rooms can be found in many of the cultural palaces, parks and clubs in the cities, where chess masters often give demonstrations and lectures on weekends and public holidays. Many people have chess sets at home, and some primary school pupils even carry the pieces in their satchels.

Xiangqi can be traced back to very early times. The earliest mention of it has been found in a book dating from 300 B.C. It became what it is today at the time of the Northern Song Dynasty (960-1127).

Like international chess, *xiangqi* is a game played by two, with 16 different pieces on each side which move in different ways. Composed of 90 positions formed by junctions of nine files and 10 ranks, the chessboard has a "river" in the middle as the boundary between the two sides. Each side moves a piece alternately, and the one who checkmates the opponent's "commander" wins the game. The 32 pieces can make a countless variety of moves. There are many similarities between *xiangqi* and international chess, the main difference being in the types and number of some of the pieces. In place of king, queen, bishop, knight, rook and pawn, *xiangqi* has commander, guard, elephant, horse, chariot, soldier and cannon, the last having no equivalent in international chess. Instead of a queen and eight pawns on each side, *xiangqi* has two guards and five soldiers.

The Chinese chess of *xiangqi* is popular in many parts of Asia. There are large numbers of enthusiasts in the Philippines, Malaysia, Thailand, Japan, Singapore, Hongkong and Macao. The First Asian Cup *Xiangqi* Tournament was held in Macao December 2-10, 1980. Future Asian Cup Tournaments will be held every other year, and there will be an invitational tournament for ranking Asian players between every two Asian Cup tournaments. With the establishment of the Asian (Chinese) Chess Federation in 1978, *xiangqi* is steadily becoming an international game.

A large number of young promising players have come to the fore in recent years. Hu Ronghua and Yang Guanlin are well-known Chinese veteran *xiangqi* players, Hu having dominated the *xiangqi* chessboard for 20 years and won 10 successive national championships. But in the 1980 national tournament he fell to 10th place and was demoted to Class B, which was listed as one of China's 10 major sports news items in that year.

Weiqi Latest archaeological discoveries and historical materials show that *weiqi* (go) originated in China more than 4,000 years ago. It was already a popular game during the Spring and Autumn and Warring States periods 2,000 years ago. *Weiqi* found its way to Japan at about the time of the Tang Dynasty (618-907). It soon won widespread popularity there which has never declined. As cultural exchanges between nations become more frequent, *weiqi* is being played in more countries than ever before. With its dissemination to countries in Europe and on the American continent, *weiqi* is well on its way to becoming an international game.

The *weiqi* board is checkered by 19 vertical lines and the same number of horizontal lines which together form a total of 361 intersections. Played with 180 black and 180 white "stones", each player in turn places a stone on an intersection, or unit of territory. The player who has encircled two or more units of territory with his stones is considered to have captured those units. The winner is the player who has more captured units and more of his own stones on the board, or simply more captured units.

After a brief decline, *weiqi* has made great headway in China in the last 30 years. The late Vice-Premier Chen Yi was a *weiqi* enthusiast. He was the first honorary chairman of the China *Weiqi* Association and did much in promoting the game and raising its standards.

In the 1950s and 1960s, Chinese *weiqi* players fell behind in skill. In the 30 games played against a visiting Japanese delegation in 1960, only two ended in favour of Chinese players and one in a draw. The gap in skill between the Chinese and Japanese players steadily narrowed in the 1970s. After 1974, the scores in matches between Chinese and Japanese players who visited each other's countries became closer every year. Sometimes Chinese players even took the lead. In the last few years, Chinese players on many occasions scored more than half of the total number of winnings. Before 1965, only a couple of Chinese players were good enough to play against

Japanese players of the eighth and ninth grades. But in recent years, more than a dozen have succeeded in defeating Japanese players of the ninth grade, among them Nie Weiping, Chen Zude, Wu Songsheng, Wang Runan and Chen Jiarui. Nie Weiping has been the most successful.

The First World Amateur Go Championship held in Tokyo in March 1979 saw 31 players participate from Europe, North America, South America, Oceania, Japan, China and south Korea — 15 countries in all. It was the first grand gathering of players in world go history. Nie Weiping won the championship title, and Chen Zude, Chen Jiarui and Kong Xiangming placed second, third and fifth respectively.

In the second world championship held in Tokyo in March 1980, a Japanese player took the title, while Chinese player Chen Jiarui was the runner-up and Liu Xiaoguang, another Chinese player, won the fourth place.

Although Chinese *weiqi* has made considerable progress, compared with *weiqi* in Japan it still lags behind in its degree of popularity and in the skill of its players. It is heartening to see that a large number of outstanding young players have come to the front. In the 1980 National Tournament of Chess Games, the 20-year-old Liu Xiaoguang took the men's title after successively beating famous players like Nie Weiping and Chen Zude. The women's title was won by a 17-year-old, Yang Hui. The two runners-up Ma Xiaochun and Kong Xiangming were also young players.

In the 1981 World Amateur Go Championship held in Japan, the champion title was won by Shao Zhenzhong, a Chinese player, who also received the rank of "seventh grade" amateur player. The Chinese player Ma Xiaochun was the runner-up.

Chinese-Style Wrestling Wrestling has been a favourite sport among China's various nationalities since ancient times. Chinese-style wrestling has its own distinct national features. Known as *jiaoli* (match of strength) or *jiaodi* (match at close quarters), wrestling was a principal part of military training in the Zhou Dynasty of the 11th century B.C. Later, it was widely practised among the people as well as in the palace. A wooden comb decorated with a coloured picture of a wrestling match was unearthed in 1975 from a tomb of the Qin Dynasty (221-207 B.C.) in Hubei Province. The picture depicts two contesting wrestlers and a referee, conveying the excitement of the match. The grandeur of the occasion is also depicted in the curtains and ribbons that hang above the arena.

Chinese wrestling found its way to Japan in the Tang Dynasty. In the Song Dynasty, when its name was changed to *xiangpu*, there were already fairly well established rules and regulations. In the Qing Dynasty (1644-1911), the name *xiangpu* was changed to *shuaijiao*. Wrestling was popular among the people, and a wrestling school was established for the training of palace guards.

Since the founding of New China, wrestling has developed considerably as a sport, particularly in rural areas and in areas inhabited by minority nationalities. Xinxian County in Shanxi Province is known as the "home of wrestling". Following a nationwide wrestling contest held in Tianjin in 1953 at the Nationalities Sports Meet, national wrestling competitions have been held frequently and wrestling has been included at all National Games.

In Chinese-style wrestling, wrestlers are divided into classes according to their weight and contests are held in a circular arena nine metres in diameter. Unlike international wrestling, formal Chinese matches require wrestlers to wear a short-sleeved jacket with an open front and a cotton waistband. A combatant can hold his opponent by any part of the body, including the jacket and the waistband, but not his pants. Tripping is permitted. Victory is gained when any part of the opponent's body above the knee touches the ground. A match is composed of three bouts, each lasting three minutes. The method of scoring is: A contestant scores three points when he causes any part of his opponent's body to touch the ground while he himself remains standing. Two points are scored in his favour if he succeeds in carrying his opponent on his shoulder or lifting him off the ground until the opponent's buttocks are higher than his chest and the opponent loses his ability to manoeuvre. The attacker wins one point if he throws his opponent off balance but only makes his hand, elbow or knee touch the ground. No point is scored if both combatants fall to the ground and it is impossible to make out which one fell first or which one is on top.

Mongolian wrestling, pursued by people of China's Mongolian nationality, is characterized by the bulk and enormous strength of the wrestlers. They are particularly skilled in employing such tactics as side kicks, twisting and leg trips. Victory is decided by one bout only and there are no division of weight classes and no limit on time or the size of the arena.

Traditional Sports of Minority Nationalities The Chinese government encourages the development of the traditional sports of minority nationalities, such as:

Mongolian horsemanship and archery. The vast grasslands and pastures in Inner Mongolia provide good natural conditions for equitation, which is a favourite sport of the people of Inner Mongolia both old and young, men and women. Grand horse races are held at the yearly Nadam Fair, a Mongolian traditional festival. Weddings, temple fairs and other festivals are often celebrated by holding horse races and archery competition. Even at ordinary times, when friends meet they like to spend part of their time together practising horse racing. Mongolian children begin to ride horseback when they are five or six. By the time they reach their teens, they are already good riders able to perform acrobatics on horseback. Show-jumping is an item that draws large crowds. Riders from Inner Mongolia invariably excel in equitation contests which have been included at all sports meets held in China since 1952.

Another traditional Mongolian sport is archery. The Inner Mongolian archery team has on many occasions won both first and second places in men's and women's group contests at national competitions. Some of China's best archers are from Inner Mongolia.

Sheep-chase in Xinjiang. Horse racing is also a favourite sport among the Uygur, Kazak and other minority nationalities in the pastoral areas of the Xinjiang Uygur Autonomous Region. The most exciting event at the New Year and other festivals, however, is the sheep-chase race. A slaughtered sheep is placed at a prearranged spot along the course of a race. The winner is the one who picks up the sheep and reaches the finishing line without letting another rider take it from him.

Horse and yak races of the Tibetans. At the annual harvest festival, the Tibetans put on their best clothes and celebrate it with singing and dancing and traditional horse and yak races. The yak race is a contest of speed. The yaks are decorated with big red flowers and beautiful saddles. The one who reaches the finishing line first wins the race.

Wrestling among the various nationalities in Yunnan. Wrestling is popular among all the minority nationalities in Yunnan Province. At the Torch Festival of the Yi people, the celebrations always include a wrestling competition. Wrestling matches are also held during work breaks and on holidays. Men of all ages, from children to elderly people, participate enthusiastically. There is no division of classes by weight and time limit. The young, inexperienced wrestlers usually enter the field first. The victor of a match remains to compete with the next contestant until he is defeated.

The annual dragon-boat race is another lively sport among the minority people living in Yunnan and Guangxi.

Korean springboard and swing. The springboard, a traditional sport of China's Korean nationality, is performed by two girls standing at either end of a seesaw plank of four or five metres in length. The momentum of the fall from a jump of one of the girls sends the other leaping into the air. The performers compete for the height reached and the feats performed in mid-air.

The swing is also a favourite sport of women of the Korean nationality. Everybody, from little girls to grandmothers, likes to make merry on the swing. Competitions are often held on festival days.

Shooting and horse riding of the Oroqen people. Inhabiting the dense forests of the Greater and Lesser Hinggan Mountains in northeast China, the Oroqen people are good hunters. Shooting and horse riding are a part of the life of both grown-ups and children. Ge Weilie, the 16-year-old son of an Oroqen hunter, won the title in the small-bore rifle 40-round standing event at the First National Games. Chosen to represent China on the national team, he distinguished himself as a "crack shot" in many international competitions.

Archery among the Xibe people. The Xibe people are an ancient tribe of hunters. After the bow and arrow lost their significance as a military weapon and a tool of production, arrow shooting became a popular folk sport among these people. There are frequent archery competitions. Two of China's ace archers Ru Guang, a young man, and Guo Meizhen, a young woman, are both of Xibe nationality. The excellent scores they have achieved at national and international competitions have attracted attention both in China and abroad.

4. COMPETITIVE SPORTS

Track and Field Few people — with limited skills — took up track and field athletics before liberation. At the 11th Olympic Games in 1936, one Chinese, Fu Baolu, a pole-vaulter, managed to make the finals, but between 1936 and 1948, only seven national records were renewed.

With the extensive development of sports after the founding of New China, the skills of athletes in track and field steadily improved. In 1957, Zheng Fengrong broke the women's high jump world record by clearing 1.77 metres. By 1958, Chinese athletes had bettered all the track and field records of old China. In 1964 alone, 43 athletes on 47 occasions smashed 19 national records, three of which were the world's second or third best achievements of that year. Chen Jiaquan, a man athlete, finished 100 metres in 10 seconds in 1965, which equalled the world record at the time. Cui Lin's time of 13.5

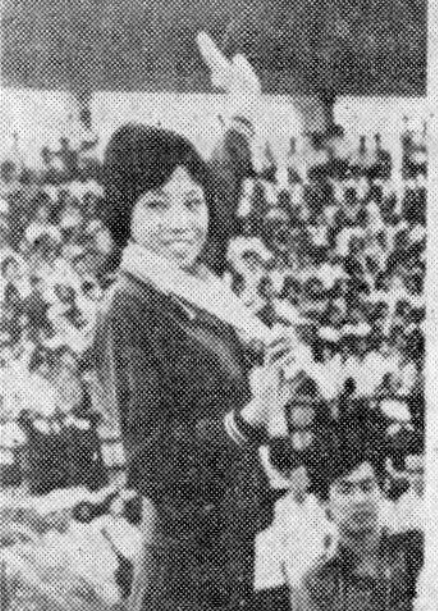
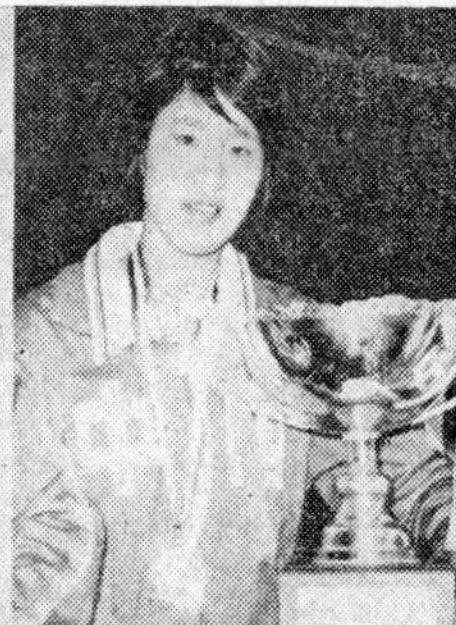
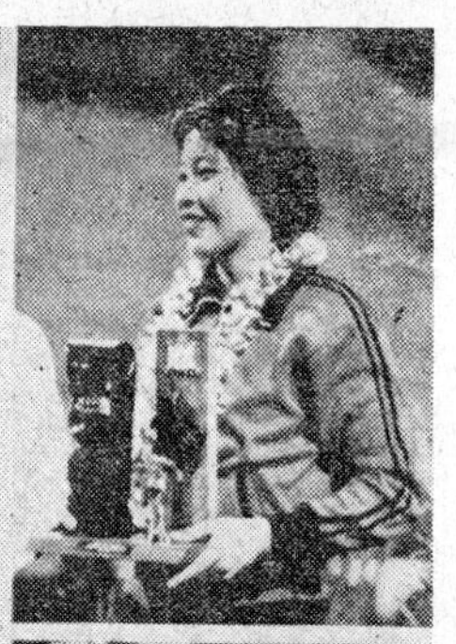
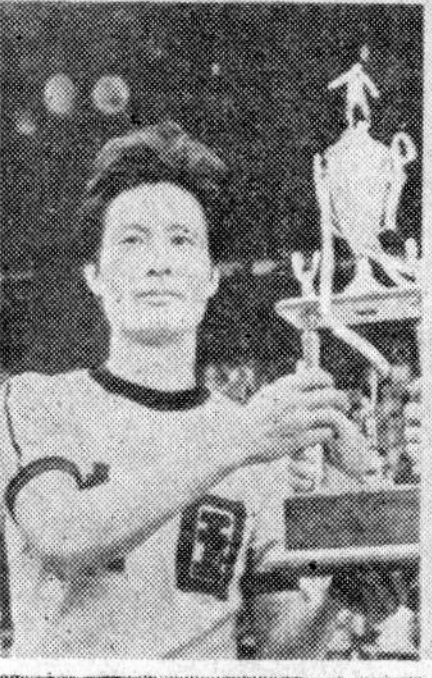
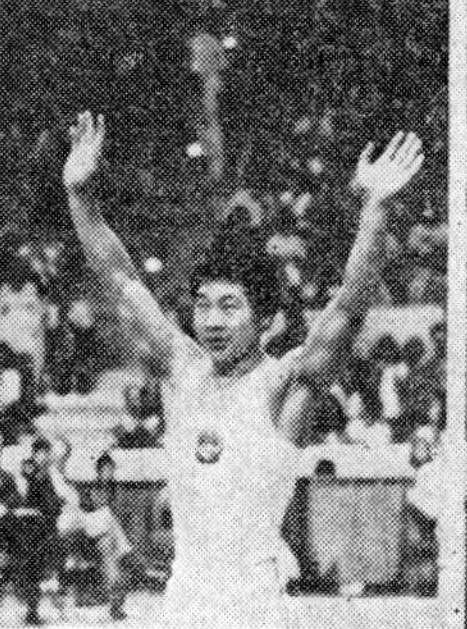
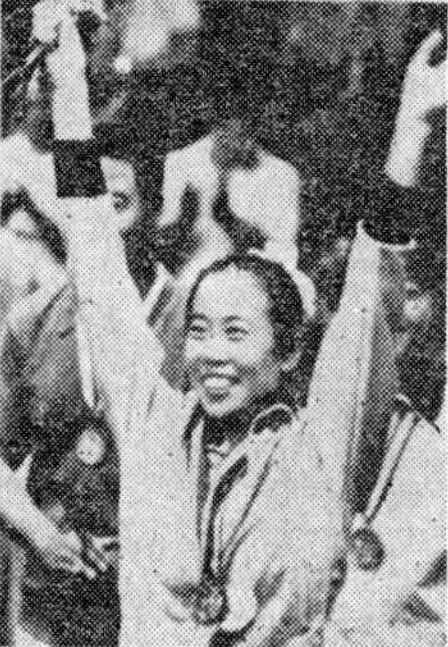
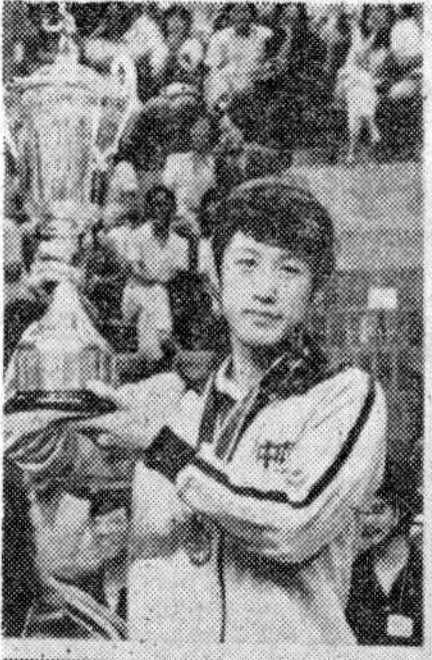
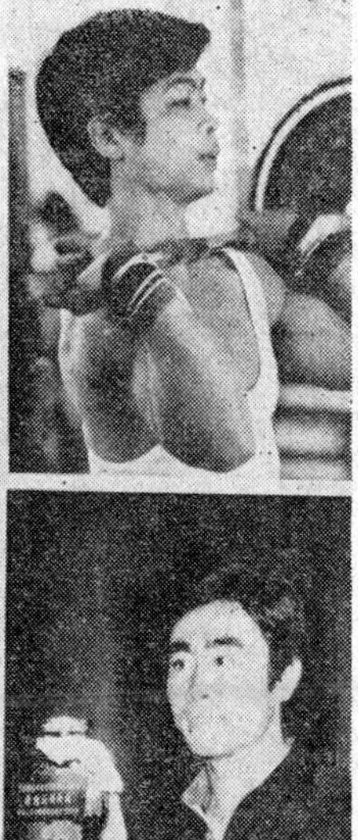
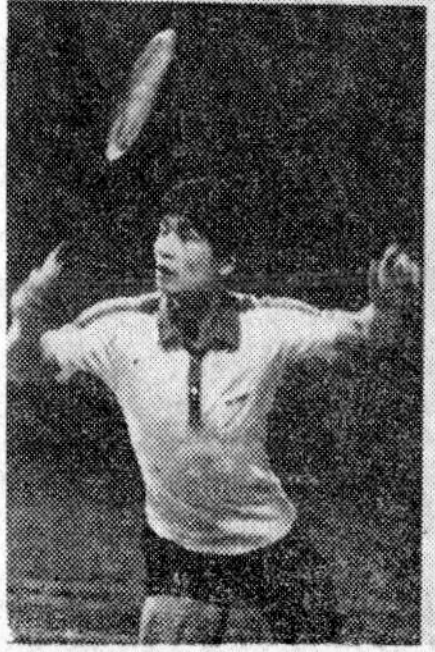

The 10 Best Athletes of 1980 selected by a nationwide poll: *Upper row, from left*: Chen Xiaoxia, Lang Ping and Liang Weifen; *second row, from left*: Rong Zhihang, Li Yuejiu and Li Cuiling; *third row, from left*: Guo Yaohua and Wu Shude; and *fourth row, from left*: Han Jian and Zou Zhenxian.

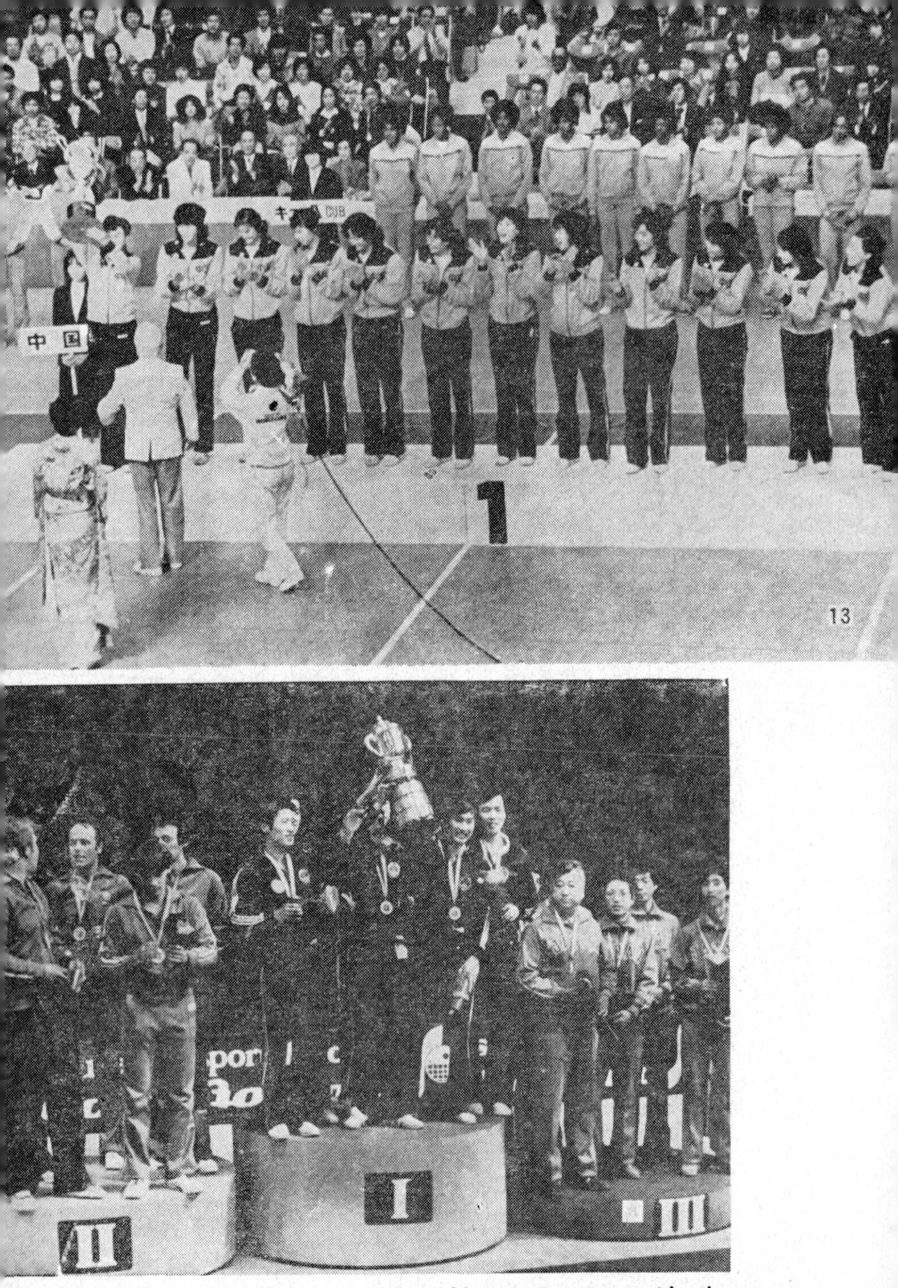

The Chinese men's table tennis team with the Swaythling Cup after winning the men's team event at the 36th World Table Tennis Championships.

he Chinese women's volley-all team, winner at the Third Vorld Cup Women's Volleyball ournament, receives the World Cup and other awards from aul Libaud, President of the édération Internationale de Volley-Ball.

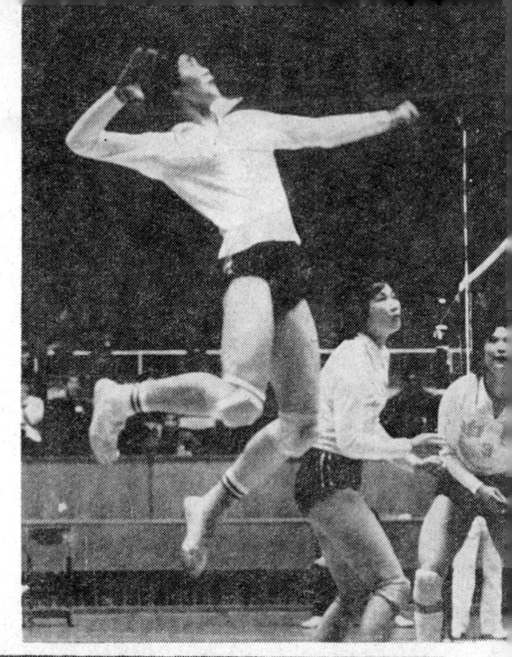

Lang Ping, the famous spiker of the Chinese women's volley-ball team, hammers the ball over the net.

Chinese players rejoice over their ictory after defeating the Japanese eam 3:2 at the Third World Cup Vomen's Volleyball Tournament.

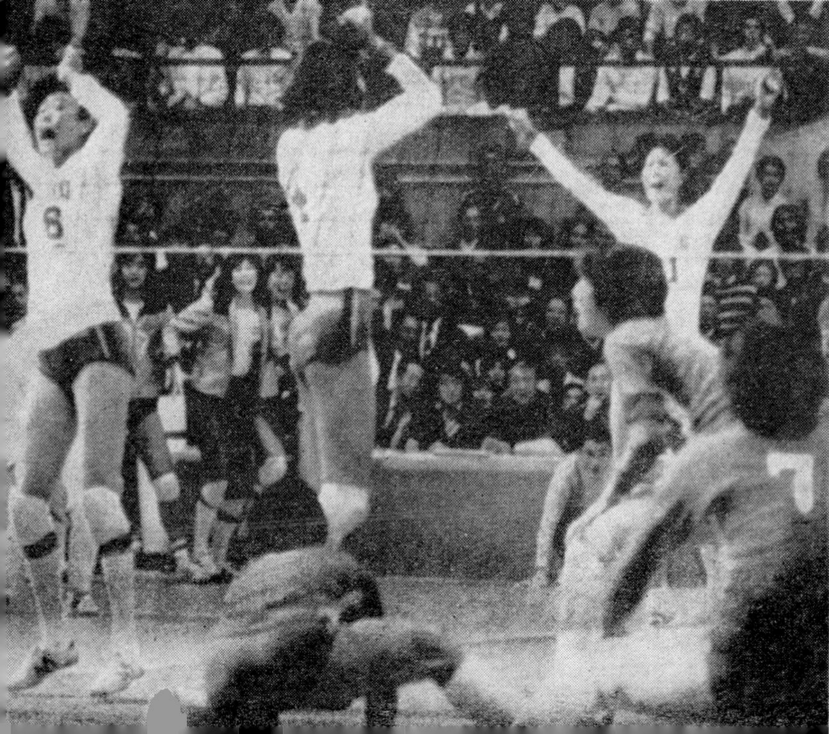

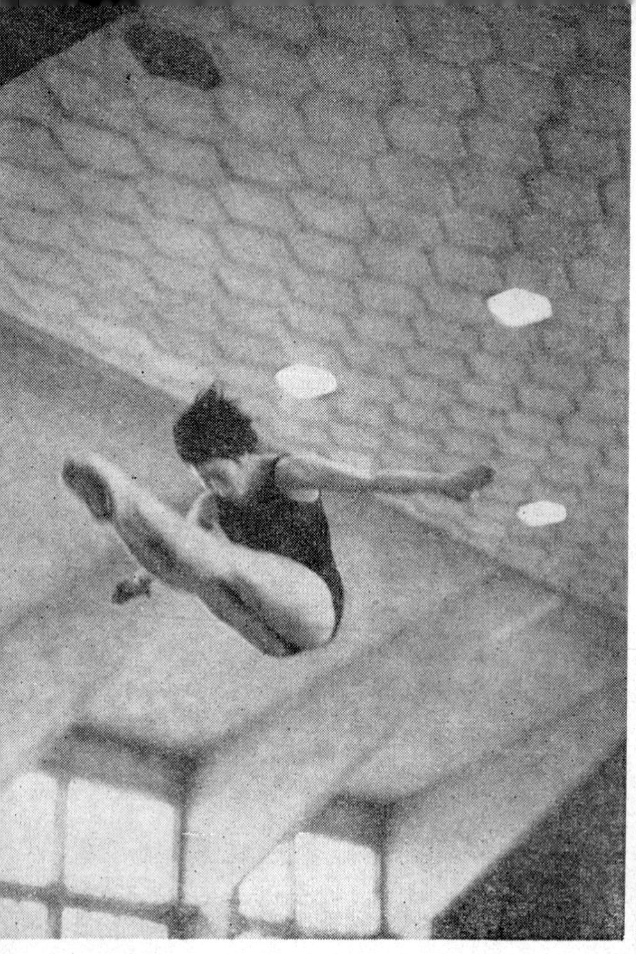

The famous Chinese woman diver Chen Xiaoxia won the women's platform event with an overwhelming margin at the Second World Cup Diving Championships held in 1981.

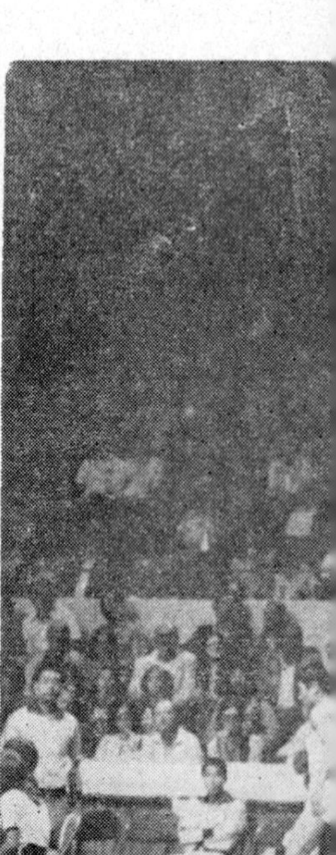

Chinese gymnasts Li Xiaoping (*right*) and Li Yuejiu (*lower*) won gold medals respectively for the pommel horse and free exercise at the 21st World Gymnastics Championships.

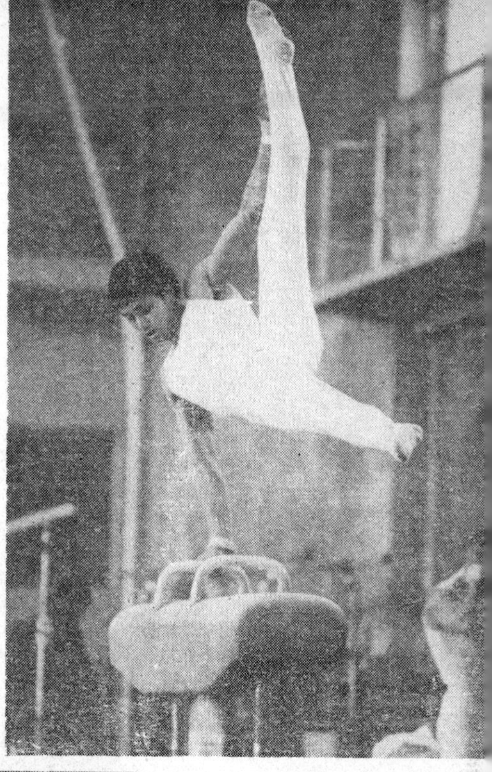

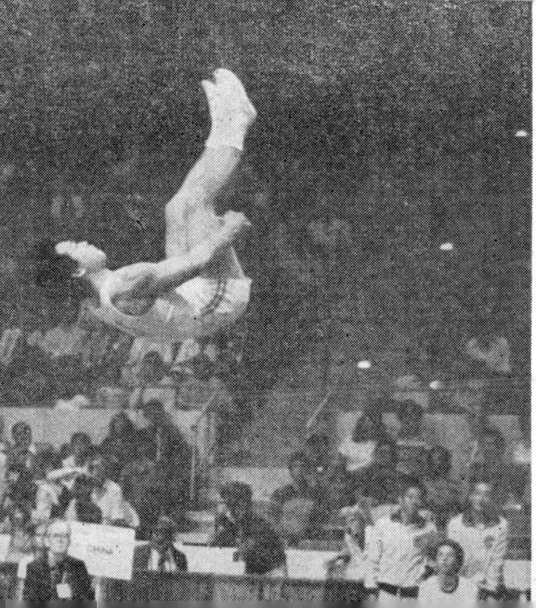

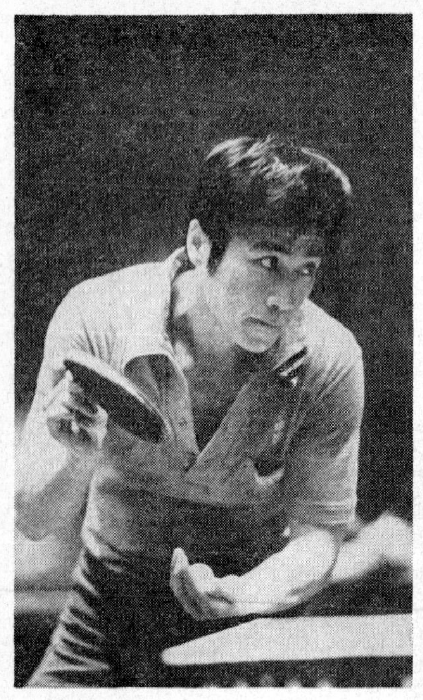

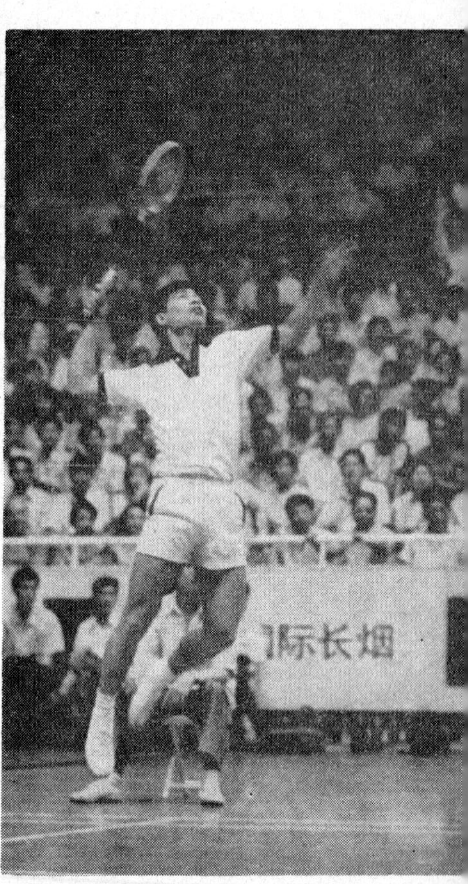
际长烟

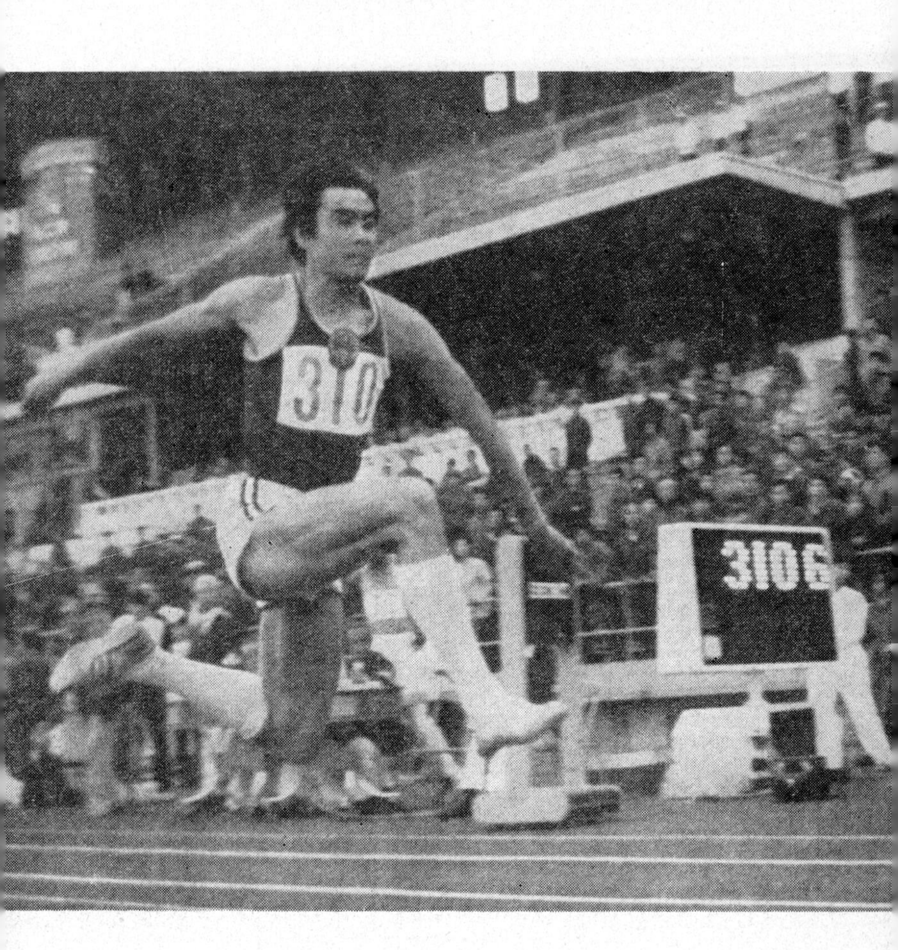

Three top Chinese athletes in action: table tennis player Guo Yaohua (*upper left*), badminton player Han Jian (*middle*) and triple jumper Zou Zhenxian (*upper right*).

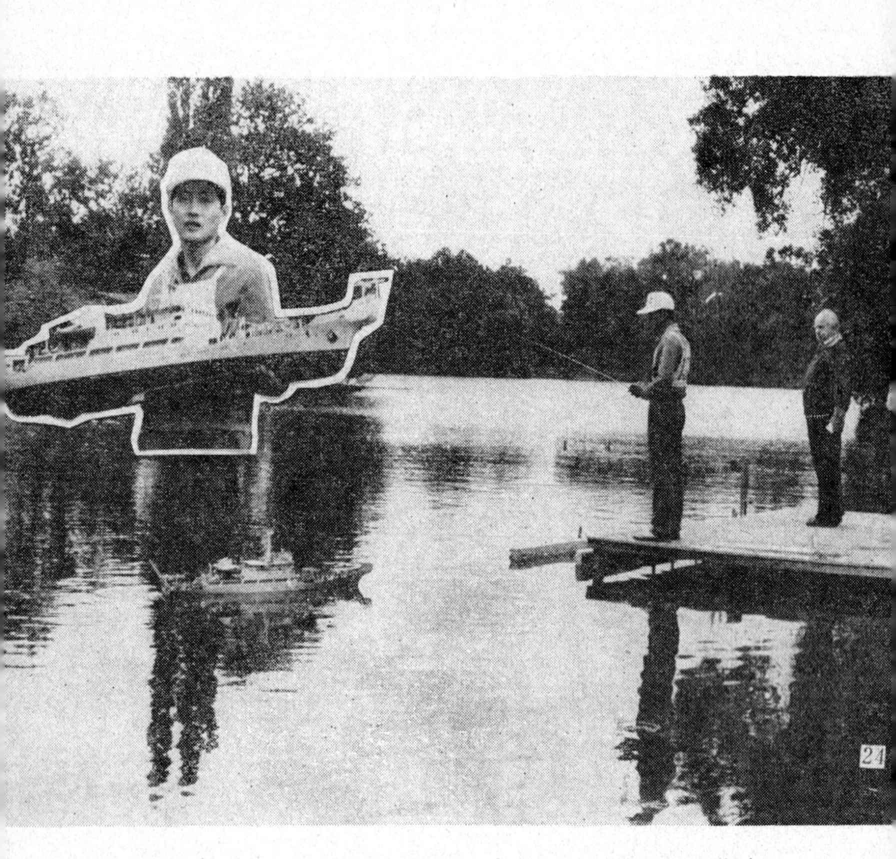

Wei Yuming won the champion title in the radio-controlled F2B event at the Second World Model Ship Championships.

seconds for the men's 110-metre hurdles was the world's best that year. Chinese athletes achieved world-class performances in men's triple jump, the marathon, women' 80-metre hurdles, high jump, long jump, shot put and discus. By that year, Chinese track and field reached its highest level of development, with 18 athletes in 11 events ranking among the world's top 10. In November 1970, Ni Zhiqin broke the men's high jump world record of that time by clearing 2.29 metres.

In recent years, China's track and field sports once again made rapid recovery and progress following the decade of the "cultural revolution". At the Eighth Asian Games in Bangkok in December 1978, Chinese athletes took the largest member of gold medals by winning 12 first places, together with 12 second places and 13 third places, in a total of 39 events. Twelve of them broke eight Asian Games records and equalled one.

In 1979, Chinese athletes also did well in both domestic and international tournaments. Twenty-six national records were bettered by 59 athletes and 7 teams on 87 occasions. At the Asian Track and Field Meet held in Japan, athletes from China smashed Asian records in men's triple jump and javelin and women's discus and pentathlon.

The year 1980 saw the best results obtained by Chinese athletes in more than 10 years. Six new Asian records were set by 8 athletes on 13 occasions, and 17 national records were improved on 42 occasions by 26 athletes (18 men and 8 women) and 2 relay teams. At a dozen or so major international competitions held in China and abroad, Chinese athletes won 34 gold medals.

Between January and March 1981, Chinese athletes scored 2 firsts and 6 second places in the international track and field tournaments in New Zealand, Kuwait, France and Japan. In the international marathon race held in April in Shanghai, Chinese runners took both the men's and women's first and second places. At the Fourth Asian Track and Field Meet in Tokyo in June, the Chinese team captured 11 gold, 4 silver and 2 bronze medals and broke 4 Asian records. Zhu Jianhua, who cleared the bar at 2.30 metres, was elected the best sportsman. Zou Zhenxian's triple jump of 17.34 metres was one of the best world results achieved in the first half of 1981. Twelve Chinese athletes (five more than on the previous occasion) were elected to represent Asia at the World Cup Athletic Championships to be held in Rome.

Despite the tremendous progress made by the Chinese athletes in recent years, they still have a long way to go to reach world advanced levels in most events. The development has been uneven. They have done better in field than track events, and women athletes have done better than men athletes. What they need in particular are advanced methods of training and more experience in international competitions.

Weightlifting Although lifting stone weights and blocks as an exercise has been popular among the Chinese people for more than 2,000 years, in the old China few people took part in weightlifting as a competitive sport and the standard was low. As weightlifting has become steadily more popular in New China, continuous improvement has been made in technique and performance. At the First National Weightlifting Competitions that took place in May 1955, all the pre-liberation national records were smashed. And it was at the Sino-Soviet Friendly Weightlifting Contests held in Shanghai in June 1956 that Chen Jingkai broke the world bantamweight clean and jerk record and thus put an end to the history of years in which no Chinese stood among the world record holders. In the next decade ending in 1966, 10 Chinese weightlifters — Chen Jingkai, Huang Qianghui, Zhao Qingkui, Li Jiyuan, Ye Haobo, Xiao Mingxiang, Chen Manlin, Ji Fayuan, Liu Dianwu and Deng Guoyin — shattered 11 clean and jerk, snatch, and press world records on 31 occasions in the bantamweight, featherweight, lightweight, middleweight and light heavyweight classes. Chen Jingkai made a name for himself in China and abroad by breaking world records nine times.

Following the period of standstill after 1966, most sports activities were not resumed until 1972. As skills gradually improved, encouraging results have been achieved in recent years. Between 1976 and 1980, among the young weightlifters of the 52-kg and 56-kg classes, 5 broke 4 world youth records on 15 occasions, and 2 broke 2 world adult records on 3 occasions.

In 1976, Cai Juncheng twice smashed the world youth snatch record of the 52 kg-class by lifting 100.5 and 101 kilogrammes. The world 52 kg-class youth records for clean and jerk and for total points were broken four times by Chen Weiqiang in 1977 — 125.5 kilogrammes and 127.5 kilogrammes for clean and jerk at the Eighth Asian Weightlifting Championships, and 128 kilogrammes for clean and jerk and 227.5 kilogrammes for total points at the China-Pakistan Friendly Weightlifting Competitions held in Guangzhou. On the latter occasion, Liu Hangyuan bettered the 56 kg-world youth record with a clean and jerk of 138 kilogrammes.

At the 1978 National Weightlifting Competitions, Wu Shude's snatch of 105.5 kilogrammes broke the 52 kg-class world youth record. In a contest with the West

German weightlifting team, Chen Weiqiang improved the 56 kg-class world youth record with a clean and jerk of 141 kilogrammes.

Chinese weightlifters continued to perform well in 1979, with 3 athletes breaking 4 world records and world youth records on 8 occasions. Chen Weiqiang began to compete in the adult group that year and broke the 56-kg clean and jerk world records with 151.5 and 153 kilogrammes respectively at the national weightlifting championships and the 33rd World Weightlifting Championships — becoming the first Chinese weightlifter to rejoin the ranks of world record holders after an absence of more than 10 years. In the same year, Wu Shude successively broke five world youth records. His snatch of 107.5 and 108 kilogrammes and his total of 235 kilogrammes at the Fifth World Youth Weightlifting Championships and the Fourth National Games exceeded the 52 kg-class world youth records, and his snatch of 110 kilogrammes and his total of 237.5 kilogrammes at the 33rd World Weightlifting Championships again set new world youth records and won the world title for snatch for himself and the first gold medal for China in world weightlifting championships. At the Fourth National Games, Zhang Yaoxin bettered the 52 kg-class world youth record with a clean and jerk of 130.5 kilogrammes.

In 1980, one world record was smashed and 14 national records bettered by 18 weightlifters on 35 occasions. Wu Shude, the young weightlifter who had six times broken world youth records, joined the ranks of the adults. At the National Weightlifting Championships, he set a new world record for snatch in the 52-kg class with 112 kilogrammes and became the first Chinese world record breaker in that class and the 12th Chinese to set a world weightlifting record. Meanwhile, Chinese weightlifters distinguished themselves at international competitions held that year. At the Shanghai International Weightlifting Invitational Tournament in which 12 countries participated, China captured the team title, 15 gold, 12 silver and 3 bronze medals. At the First American Continental Cup Weightlifting Championships, China again won 4 first places, 5 second places and 1 third place, plus the team title.

Twelve Chinese weightlifters have broken 12 world records in 6 weight classes on 34 occasions in the years 1949-1980. These achievements will still have to be bettered to reach the world advanced levels. On the whole, Chinese weightlifters have done better in individual events of the lighter classes than in total points and the heavier classes.

Gymnastics Competitive gymnastics is new in China, having been practised only after the founding of the People's Republic. The First National Gymnastics Contest held in Beijing in 1953 was participated in by 67 gymnasts, who competed only in a limited number of events. Since 1955, a national contest has been held every year in which an ever-increasing number of gymnasts with ever-increasing skills compete.

In 1958, China competed for the first time in the World Gymnastics Championships (the 14th) with the women's team placing seventh, the men's team 11th. At the 15th World Gymnastics Championships in 1962, Chinese gymnasts gave a better account of themselves, winning the fourth place in the men's team event and the sixth place in the women's team event, and the third place on the pommel horse.

At the First Games of the New Emerging Forces held

in Djakarta in 1963, the Chinese men's and women's teams were both runners-up in the team event. In the men's and women's all-round events and 10 individual events, Chinese gymnasts won eight titles. The 17-year-old newcomer Wang Weijian alone captured four titles in the women's all-round, free exercise, balance beam and vaulting horse. At the First Asian Games of the New Emerging Forces held in Phnom Penh in 1966, Chinese gymnasts won the men's and women's team titles and championships in both the men's and women's all-round events with some highly difficult manoeuvres rarely seen in international competition.

In 14 events at the Seventh Asian Games held in Tehran in 1974, the Chinese team scored eight first places — including the men's and women's team titles — and seven second places.

At the Eighth Asian Games held in Bangkok in 1978, Chinese gymnasts collected 10 gold medals, capturing the men's and women's team titles and all the first three places in the men's and women's all-round events.

The Chinese men's team was placed fifth and women's team fourth at the 20th World Gymnastics Championships in December 1979 in Fort Worth, Texas, in the United States. The world title for the uneven bars was won by the 15-year-old Chinese girl Ma Yanhong with a series of difficult, new and steadily and beautifully executed moves. After an absence of 17 years — since the 15th World Gymnastics Championships in 1962 — Chinese gymnasts fully demonstrated their skills on their return to international competitions in 1979 and were qualified to compete at the 1980 Olympic Games.

In 1980, the Chinese gymnastics team again scored a series of victories in international competitions, winning praise both in China and abroad. In the invitational tournament held in Hartford, Connecticut, in the United States, in August, the Chinese team carried off nine champion titles: men's and women's team titles, women's all-round and six of the 10 men's and women's individual titles. The Japanese national team which was champion for 10 times in succession at the World Championships and the Olympic Games was defeated by the Chinese men's team, while the Chinese women's team captured almost all the titles. Also in August, at the Ninth Women's World Gymnastics Meet held in Antibes, France, Jiang Wei and Wu Wenli, two 12-year-old Chinese girls, won the all-round and balance beam titles respectively. The Fifth Gymnastics World Cup was held in October in Toronto, Canada, in which 11 countries participated. Two gold medals were won by Chinese gymnasts — Li Yuejiu on the parallel bars and Huang Yubin on the rings. In the 1980 Chunichi Cup international tournament held in Nagoya in November that year, China's Li Cuiling captured the women's all-round, vaulting horse and balance beam titles; Tang Xiaoli was the all-round runner-up and champion on the uneven bars and in the free exercise. In the competition on the pommel horse, Li Xiaoping took the championship after defeating all his rivals with a number of perfectly executed difficult feats.

The year 1981 saw Chinese gymnasts take 66 first places in international competitions. At the 21st World Gymnastics Championships held in Moscow in November that year, the Chinese team won second place in the women's team event and third place in the men's team event. The gold medals for the men's floor exercise and pommel horse went respectively to Li Yuejiu and Li Xiaoping, the silver medals for the rings, uneven bars and balance beam went respectively to Huang Yubin, Ma Yanhong and Chen Yongyan, and the bronze medal for the uneven bars went to Wu Jiani.

Sports Acrobatics In China, sports acrobatics began to develop as a competitive event according to international rules only after its introduction to the country in 1956 and a national competition held in 1957. The skills of the Chinese sports acrobats have since steadily improved. The Chinese Association of Sports Acrobatics joined the International Federation of Sports Acrobatics in December 1979. In September 1980, Chinese acrobats made their debut in the World Championships in Sports Acrobatics (the fourth, held in Poznan, Poland), in which they carried off 11 bronze medals, winning 5 third places in 7 all-around events and 6 third places in 14 single exercises.

Chinese sports acrobatics has developed a distinct national style, a style characterized by combining acrobatics with gymnastics and dance. In international competitions, the Chinese gymnasts have given full display to their national characteristics, performed moves involving a high degree of difficulty and created human-figure compositions with close coordination. They have received favourable comments from friends of all countries.

Swimming The five-star red flag of the People's Republic of China was hoisted for the first time in an international sports competition in 1953 at the Fourth World Youth Festival when Chinese swimmer Wu Chuanyu won first place in the men's 100-metre backstroke. After the founding of the People's Republic and with the encouragement of Chairman Mao Zedong, swimming became one of the most popular sports and swimming skills have developed accordingly, especially since China's long coastline and innumerable lakes and rivers provide such good natural conditions for swimming.

The First National Swimming Competitions were held in New China in 1952. By 1954, swimmers in China had broken all the pre-liberation records and begun to move towards advanced world levels. Between 1957 and 1960, three Chinese swimmers, Qi Lieyun, Mu Xiangxiong and Mo Guoxiong, bettered the men's 100-metre breaststroke world record five times. China's record in the men's 100-metre freestyle was also among the world's best. More successes were achieved in 1965. Zhou Tongwen, Bu Zigang and Dong Rentian ranked among the world's first 10 swimmers respectively in the 100-metre freestyle, 100-metre breaststroke and 200-metre breaststroke. Four other swimmers finished the 100-metre breaststroke in 1 minute 11 seconds, the 1960 world record set by Mo Guoxiong.

Renewed progress had been made in recent years. In 1979, 34 swimmers and four teams broke 25 national records on 140 occasions, and in 1980, 24 swimmers and five teams improved 26 national records (13 men's and 13 women's) on 116 occasions. Wang Lin's national record of 1 minute 4.5 seconds in the men's 100-metre breaststroke and Liang Weifen's record of 1 minute 12.84 seconds in the women's 100-metre breaststroke were both placed the world's 18th in 1980.

Chinese swimmers won two first places and five second places in the international swimming contests held in New Zealand, Australia and Britain in January and February 1981. But on the whole, China still lags far behind the leading swimming countries in the world.

Diving Unknown as a competitive sport before 1949, diving has made rapid progress in China since the first nationwide diving competitions held in 1952. At the Seventh Asian Games in 1974, the Chinese diving team took the first places in all the four events. Again at the Eighth Asian Games in 1978, all the gold and silver medals in the four events went to Chinese divers. Some of the difficult dives they performed already measure up to advanced international levels. All the seven Chinese divers competing at the World University Games held in Mexico in 1979 won places among the best six in each event. Seventeen-year-old Chen Xiaoxia won top honours in the women's 10-metre platform diving competition after defeating the world champion of 1978, Irina Kalinina of the Soviet Union.

In international competitions in 1980, Chinese divers once again showed their outstanding skills. In the contest between Chinese and American divers held in April 1980 in Columbus, Ohio, the Chinese divers taking three of the four titles, came off with a victory of 45-43 for both the men's and women's teams. The American team, one of the strongest in the world, was composed of the best U.S. divers recently selected through national eliminations. Four months later, the American team paid a return visit to China. The two teams each took two titles, and the Chinese team won 68-65 in total score.

The Chinese diving team taking part in the Martini International Diving Competition, a world-level contest, held in London in November 1980, captured three first places and one second place in the four events and won the team title with a total score of 45, surpassing the teams from the United States, the Soviet Union and the German Democratic Republic. The women's platform diving event was won by Chen Xiaoxia, and the men's springboard diving event by Li Kongzheng. The Chinese girl Shi Meiqin captured the women's springboard title, eclipsing Irina Kalinina of the Soviet Union, the women's springboard diving champion at the 22nd Olympic Games in Moscow.

Competing at the New Zealand Summer Games in which 28 countries and regions took part in January 1981, Chinese divers won top places in all four diving events: Jin Weidong in the men's springboard event, Zeng Xilong in the men's platform event and Du Huiying in both the women's springboard and platform events. In June that year, at the Second World Cup Diving Championships held in Mexico, Shi Meiqin won the women's 3-metre springboard event; Li Hongping, the men's platform event; and Chen Xiaoxia, the women's platform event.

Basketball The Soviet national basketball team visited China at the end of 1950 and played 33 matches against Chinese teams. The latter lost all the matches by a big margin, the worst score being 191:35. This gives some indication of the poor foundation and low technical level of basketball immediately after the founding of the People's Republic.

Today, basketball has become one of the most favourite sports of the people in both the cities and rural areas. It has an extensive popular base, and in 30 and more years, Chinese basketball players have rapidly improved their skills.

From 1953 to 1957, Chinese basketball teams played in a total of 283 international matches, scoring 163 wins, 7 draws and 113 losses. In 1957, the Chinese teams defeated the Yugoslav and some other European teams and began to show their prowess.

Between 1958 and 1960, Chinese basketball approached world advanced level in skills. In the 196 international matches played during this period, the Chinese men's teams scored 114 wins and 7 draws. The women's teams achieved 90 wins and 9 draws in 135 international matches. In 1958, the Beijing women's basketball team beat the Czechoslovak team, the third best in the World Championships, by 64-54, and in 1959 the Chinese national women's team beat the Hungarian national team by 59-38, and finished in 2 draws against the Bulgarian team, the runner-up in the World Women's Basketball Championships. In the same year, the Chinese men's team triumphed over the Hungarian team by 73-70 and 65-60 and over the powerful Czechoslovak and Bulgarian teams by 82-64 and 86-77 respectively.

In the years from 1961 to 1965, more headway was made in improving the technical level. The visiting Soviet national champion team — the Armed Forces Men's Basketball Team (with eight national team members) — lost to the team of the Chinese People's Liberation Army's Beijing units 55-60, and won a narrow victory over the Chinese People's Liberation Army Team, 66-65, in 1962. At the First Games of the New Emerging Forces held in Djakarta in 1963, the Chinese men's and women's teams both captured the team titles by winning all the matches. The Polish men's basketball team, winner of sixth place at the 18th Olympic Games, visited China in 1964 to play five matches. The Chinese teams won four of them. In the same year, the Chinese women's team was placed first in the competitions held in France between China, France, Romania and Hungary.

Basketball in China suffered a decline in the decade after 1966. No young talents were trained during this period to take the place of the veterans. There have been some signs of recovery only in recent years when Chinese basketball teams began to gain some successes in international competitions. After the restoration of China's legitimate seat in the Fédération Internationale de Basketball Amateur in 1974, China has been taking part in an increasing number of international matches. The Chinese women's basketball team captured the championship title for the first time in the Asian competitions in 1976. In the Eighth and Ninth Asian Men's Basketball Championships in 1975 and 1977, the Chinese men's basketball team succeeded in winning the championship on both occasions. The Chinese team managed to beat the south Korean team 91-77 and the Japanese national team 95-76 in the basketball matches at the Eighth Asian Games in 1978. The Chinese team won a narrow victory over the Japanese team again in 1979 at the 10th Asian Championships capturing the Asian championship for the fourth time in succession and qualifying itself to represent Asia at the 22nd Olympic Games of 1980.

The men's basketball team of the Chinese People's Liberation Army (the August 1st Team) has also been doing quite well in matches against home and foreign teams. In early 1979, it notched two wins in Beijing, 104-96 and 72-69, against the joint team of American universities. In August the same year, in a match against the 1978 American professional basketball champion, the "Bullet" team, the August 1st Team lost only by eight points. The Chinese army team defeated the Italian team at the 27th International Military Sports Council (CISM) Basketball Championships held in Fayetteville, the United States, in 1980 and rose to the third place from their fourth place showing the year before.

The Chinese women's basketball team finished 10th in the qualifying tournament in Bulgaria in May 1980 for the 22nd Olympic Games. In the second stage of the tournament, the Chinese women cagers displayed their potential when they outplayed the Cuban team, the 5th in the 21st Olympic Games, by 85-78 and the Italian team, the 6th in the 21st Olympic Games, by 62-60, but lost to the Bulgarian team, the runner-up of the 21st Olympic Games, by one point. The Chinese men's basketball team won top honours at the Sixth Asian Youth Basketball Championships held in Bangkok in December 1980 after dethroning the Philippine team, the winning team in the previous five championships. The Chinese women's team was the runner-up at the Eighth Asian Championships held in Hongkong, but in the final, it lost to the south Korean team by an astounding margin of 33 points.

The August 1st men's basketball team competing at the First Asian Club Championships in Hongkong in March 1981 carried off the title without a single loss. Two of its players, Guo Yonglin and Ma Lianbao, shared the best-player prize. Both the boys' and girls' basketball teams from China emerged as victors at the International Basketball Tournament for School Teams held in Belgium in April that year. In the 1981 International Women's Basketball Invitational Tournament which took place in Jinan, Shandong Province, in May of that year, the Chinese women's team came in first with six wins in seven matches, over a field which included the Yugoslav team, the third place winner at the Olympic Games; and the Canadian and Australian teams, the third and fourth in the last World Women's Basketball Championships.

To improve their technique and to catch up with advanced world levels, what the Chinese players need most is intensified training, including basic training and training in physical development, cultivating a stubborn fighting spirit and developing a Chinese style of play.

Volleyball The six-man volleyball became popular in China only after the founding of the People's Republic, and the standard then was rather low. A guiding principle of "initiative, speed and flexibility" was put forward in 1955 for intensifying training and raising skills in accordance with the characteristics of the Chinese players. China competed for the first time on the world arena in 1956, at the men's third and women's second world volleyball championships held in Paris. The Chinese men's team placed ninth, and women's team sixth. In 1957, a slogan for training was raised: "All-round skills and varied tactics." Since 1963, the Chinese volleyball team adopted a new method of training, which emphasized higher intensity. In the international competitions of that year, the Chinese volleyball team foiled the Japanese men's team, the fifth in the world, and the Japanese women's team, one of the best in the world, and won both the men's and women's titles at the First Games of the New Emerging Forces. In 1964, the Chinese volleyball team, while learning from the advanced skills of the other countries, assimilated its own experience and achieved satisfactory results by training with higher intensity according to the principle that "training should be hard, strict and geared to actual competition". The Chinese players learned from the strong points of other players, blazed a trail of their own and cultivated a style of all-round skills, high speed, high reach, flexibility and precision. Compared with basketball and football players, Chinese volleyball players have made more rapid progress. The Chinese women volleyball players, in particular, have been in the lead in becoming a shock brigade full of drive. Chinese volleyball is striding forward by leaps and bounds towards top world level.

At the women's second and men's third volleyball World Cup held in Japan in September 1977, the Chinese women's team finished fourth, and men's team fifth. In 1978, the Chinese women's team won sixth place at the Eighth World Women's Volleyball Championships in the Soviet Union, and the men's team was seventh in the Ninth World Men's Volleyball Championships that took place in Italy.

Chinese volleyball's rapid progress was abundantly demonstrated at the Second Asian Women's Volleyball Championships in Hongkong and the Second Asian Men's Volleyball Championships in Bahrain in December 1979. The Chinese women's team, by a score of three sets to one, beat the Japanese team, the six-time champion and six-time runner-up at the World Championships and Olympic Games, and defeated the south Korean team, the bronze medal winner at the 1976 Olympic Games, in three-straight sets, to capture the crown after winning all six matches played. The Chinese men's team did the same after breaking the defence of the Japanese and south Korean teams. Both Chinese teams were qualified to compete in the 1980 Olympic Games on behalf of Asia.

The Chinese men's and women's teams saw fewer large-scale international volleyball competitions in 1980. But they did very well in some team-to-team and multi-team competitions against the world's strongest players. During its visits to Latin America and Japan, the men's team won all 22 matches it played. In its matches against the many-time champion Japanese team and the U.S. team, which is reinforced by the world's No. 1 spiker, Flora Hyman, the Chinese women's team scored respectively four wins in four matches and eight wins and one loss. In December 1980 and January 1981, the Chinese women's team participating in the ninth Schwerte international tournament and the second Bremen international tournament in West Germany finished first, winning all the four matches. The two exhibition matches included, the team won a total of 30 games without losing a single one.

Both the men's and women's teams placed first at the Asian Qualifying Tournaments for World Cup held in March 1981. At the Third World Cup women's volleyball championship held in Japan in November 1981, the Chinese team carried off the title after winning all seven matches it played. It was the first world title ever won by Chinese players in the three principal ball games — basketball, volleyball and football. The Chinese men's team retained its fifth place at the Fourth World Cup men's volleyball championship also held in Japan in November.

Football The popularity of football in China grew after the birth of the People's Republic, but the technical level has not increased fast enough during the past 30 years of difficult development.

In old China, football was played only in a few large cities. Players' skills began to improve in New China but they still needed much improvement: in 1951, the Chinese People's Liberation Army team lost 1:17 and 1:9 respectively to the People's Army teams of Czechoslovakia and Bulgaria. The following year, the Chinese national team lost to the Polish team 1:7 and to the Finnish team 0:4.

Skills did begin to improve in 1954 after reforms in the organization of matches, intensified training and more international matches both in China and abroad which gave Chinese players the needed experience. In the 166 international matches played between 1954 and 1957, the Chinese teams scored 49 wins, 26 draws and 91 losses. The match against the Czechoslovak People's Army team ended in a draw. The Chinese team was victorious in the match against the Polish team.

In 1958 and 1959, the Chinese football team played two matches against the Soviet national team, the champion team at the 16th Olympic Games. Both ended in a tie. The Chinese team beat the Hungarian team 1:0 in 1959 in a tri-meet between the Chinese team, the Soviet national team and Hungary's second national team, and it placed first in matches between the four countries of China, Korea, Viet Nam and Mongolia in 1960. From 1958 to 1961, Chinese teams played in 237 international matches, winning 88, drawing 51 and losing 98. After that, as matches were irregular and training was poor, there was a decline in skill until the 1970s.

The Chinese Football Association joined the Asian Football Confederation in 1974 and was restored to its legitimate seat in the Fédération Internationale de Football Association (FIFA) in 1979.

In 1977 and 1978, 33 Chinese football teams visited 47 countries and regions, and football teams from 29 countries and regions came to China. Competitions on these occasions promoted friendship and helped improve the players' skills. In September 1977, the matches between the Chinese team and the New York Cosmos, the American professional team with world-famous stars Pelé and Beckenbauer in it, ended in one draw and one win for China. Later, when the Chinese team visited the United States, the match against the Cosmos team again finished in a draw of 1:1. At the 1978 Eighth Asian Games, the Chinese team placed third. The year 1979 saw 10 Chinese football teams going out to 16 countries and regions and 10 foreign teams coming to China. For the first time, the Chinese teams scored more wins than losses: in 83 matches, the Chinese teams registered 38 wins, 15 draws and 30 losses. Between 1977 and 1980, China sponsored three international football friendly invitational tournaments in which the Chinese team placed first twice and second once. After suffering two losses at the Olympic preliminaries (Asian-Oceanian Zone, Group 3) and the Asian Cup finals in March and September 1980, the Chinese footballers learned from their experience, intensified training and consequently made new headway. The Chinese team won five straight matches in the finals at the 12th World Cup Asian-Oceanian Zone Group 4 Qualifying Football Tournament and placed first in the group on January 4, 1981. Competing with the best teams in the other three groups for the right to represent the Asian-Oceanian Zone in the World Cup final series in Spain in 1982, the Chinese players first scored 8 wins, 1 draw and 3 losses, but was eliminated in the last match.

Although some improvements have been made, the technical level of Chinese football is still behind that of the leading football nations. The Chinese team ranks between 40th and 50th in the world, at about the same level as the weaker teams in the B Division of leading European football countries and slightly lower than some stronger teams in Asia. Chinese footballers are looking reality in the face and doing their utmost to catch up.

Table Tennis Table tennis was the pastime of a few people in the old China, and no Chinese player was known to the world. Today, China has become one of the countries in the world where table tennis is most popular and where the best players can be found.

China competed for the first time in the world championships (the 20th) in 1953. Its men's team secured 10th place in the men's first division, and its women's team the third place in the women's second division. After that, table tennis quickly developed as a popular sport. In 1958, an estimated 50 million people were playing table tennis in China. At the 25th World Table Tennis Championships in 1959, both the men's and women's teams from China finished third in the team event. Chinese player Rong Guotuan captured the men's singles title, the first world title in any sport ever taken by a Chinese. This served as an important turning point in the history of table tennis in China. A table tennis craze then appeared in this country, and table tennis as a sport has been making continuous leaps forward.

The 1960s saw Chinese table tennis enter into a period of full bloom, putting an end to the monopoly enjoyed by the Japanese players since the 1950s. The Chinese team carried off three gold, four silver and eight bronze medals at the 26th World Table Tennis Championships in 1961, and five gold, four silver and seven bronze medals at the 28th World Championships in 1965.

The Chinese team was absent from the 1967 and 1969 World Championships. At the 31st Championships in 1971, four titles were captured by veteran Chinese players who had matured as players before 1966. The Chinese team won three titles at the 32nd World Championships in 1973 and two titles at the 33rd World Championships in 1975, after fierce contention. At the 34th

World Championships held in 1977, the Chinese team secured three and a half titles.

The 35th World Table Tennis Championships was held in 1979 in Pyongyang, where the Chinese team carried off four gold medals: for the women's team event, women's singles, women's doubles and mixed doubles; four silver medals: for the men's team event, men's singles, women's doubles and mixed doubles; and seven bronze medals. Six Chinese men players and five Chinese women players were among the world's 16 best table tennis players listed by the International Table Tennis Federation in 1979.

Chinese players achieved remarkable success in the 11 important international competitions in which they participated in 1980, capturing 54 of 65 championship titles in these competitions — including all the titles in the men's and women's team events and women's singles and nine of the 11 men's singles titles, one of which was Guo Yaohua's win at the First World Cup Table Tennis Championship.

At the 36th World Table Tennis Championships held in Yugoslavia in 1981, the Chinese players captured all the titles in the seven events and all the second places in the individual events — something which had never happened before in the 55 years' history of world table tennis championships.

Beginning in 1961, the year in which Chinese players won three major world titles, China has maintained its lead in table tennis for 20 years. Previously, both Japan — a leading table tennis country for 17 years — and Hungary had won as many as six titles. In the 10 world championships in which China has participated since 1959 when Rong Guotuan won the first world title for

China, Chinese players have collected 36 of the 70 gold medals and 31 of the 50 silver, over half of the total. Up to the present, Chinese table tennis players have won world titles on 87 occasions, carrying home a total of 255 gold, silver and bronze medals.

Badminton Badminton caught on in China around 1954. The First National Badminton Championships were held in Tianjin in 1956, and from then on a national competition has been held every year.

With the return to China from overseas of Fang Kaixiang, Tang Xianhu, Chen Yuniang and Hou Jiachang in 1959, new blood was pumped into badminton in China. There was then a marked change in the method of training, technique and tactics. A new style of play was developed, characterized by "speed, ferocity, precision and flexibility". Chinese players joined the front ranks of world badminton players when they gained the upper hand in their encounters with the Indonesian team, winner of the Thomas Cup, and the Danish team, another perennial badminton power, in 1964 and 1966.

The Chinese badminton team carried off five major titles — men's and women's team titles, men's and women's singles titles and women's doubles title — at the Seventh Asian Games in 1974 and six titles in the nine individual events at the Fourth Asian Badminton Championships in 1976. In 1977, at the Second Asian Badminton Invitational Competitions, young Chinese players won top honours in three of the four events.

After the birth of the new World Badminton Federation in the spring of 1978, the Chinese team competing in the First World Badminton Championships won four of the five titles (men's and women's singles and doubles). In December the same year, at the Eighth Asian Games, the Chinese team captured three titles, but lost to Indonesia in the men's team event.

At the First World Cup Badminton Championships (team events only) and the Second World Badminton Championships (individual events only) held in Hangzhou in June 1979 under the sponsorship of the World Badminton Federation, Chinese players captured both the men's and women's team titles, and titles in the men's and women's singles and men's doubles. The match between China and the world badminton power Indonesia in Hongkong in December that year ended in favour of China, its women's team scoring 5:0 and men's team 6:3.

Another duel between the Chinese and Indonesia teams took place in Singapore in February 1980. Han Jian on the Chinese side defeated Liem Swie King, Indonesia's No. 1 seeded player and twice all-England champion, to win a crucial point for the Chinese team. The Chinese men's team notched a narrow victory 5:4 in this duel, which was considered by some people as badminton competition at its best in the world today. The Chinese women's team lost to Indonesia by 1:3. At the Fourth Asian Badminton Invitational Competitions held in Bangkok in December that year, the Chinese players took all the four men's and women's individual titles and all the first four places in the men's and women's singles.

Chinese badminton players scored remarkable successes in international competitions in 1981. In the star-studded badminton tournament of the First World Games for Non-Olympic Sports held in July, the Chinese team took four titles in the five individual events — men's singles and doubles, and women's singles and doubles. At the World's Premier Open Badminton Tournament held in London in September, Chinese players won the titles in the men's and women's singles and women's doubles, and at the Alba World Cup Badminton Championships held in Malaysia in October, they claimed the first and second places in the women's singles and the second, third and fourth places in the men's singles. Their successes have placed them among the best players in the world.

Fencing A traditional European sport which is different from the Chinese exercise with a sword, fencing was introduced into China in the mid-1950s. China participated in international competitions for the first time in 1974, at the World Fencing Championships. In the individual contests, Chinese foil player Chen Jingxi defeated Yassily Stankovich, the 1971 men's foil champion, from the Soviet Union. Two Chinese men and two women contestants entered the semi-finals at the 28th World Junior Fencing Championships in 1977.

In the 77 years of world fencing contests from 1901 to 1977, all the top places were monopolized by European contestants; Asian fencers were eliminated before they reached the finals. But at the 29th World Junior Fencing Championships held in Madrid in March 1978, the 19-year-old Chinese contestant Luan Jujie won the right to compete in the finals. In the first round of the finals, her sword-holding left arm was wounded by the Soviet opponent's broken foil. Bearing the pain stoically, she eventually put her rival to the rout. She then fought five more rounds to emerge as the runner-up in the world youth women's foil fencing. She was the first Asian girl ever to mount the podium in international fencing contests.

At the Eighth Asian Games held in December 1978, the Chinese fencing team garnered four gold medals —

by Luan Jujie and Wang Ruiji in the women's foil and sabre, by the Chinese team composed of Luan Jujie and three others in the women's foil team contest after thwarting the powerful Japanese team, and by the Chinese team in the épée team contests.

The Chinese women's team won eighth place in the foil team contest at the 35th World Fencing Championships held in Melbourne in August 1979, and Chinese contestants placed sixth among the seven best teams in the world women's foil fencing contest held in Frankfurt in March 1980.

In July 1981, the Chinese women fencer Luan Jujie again won the silver medal in the women's foil fencing at the 36th World Fencing Championships.

Archery Although the bow and arrow dates back to time immemorial, archery as a competitive sport according to modern international rules began in China only in 1959. In 1961, Zhao Suxia became the first Chinese archer to break a world record. In 1963, Li Shulan, then 18, broke five world records during a tournament to become the holder of half of the women's world individual records. Between 1961 and 1966, 13 world records (11 of which were women's) were broken by seven Chinese archers and three teams on 29 occasions.

Wang Wenjuan broke the women's 30-metre single-round world record in 1974. She was followed by Huang Shuyan, Jiang Shengling and Song Shuxian, who altogether bettered world records 10 times in three years.

Chinese archers have done even better since 1977. In that year, Song Shuxian set a new women's 70-metre single-round world record by scoring 317 points. In March 1978, Song Shuxian, Meng Fanai and Huang Shuyan broke the women's single-round world team record with a score of 3,780 points. All the men's national records were also broken when 14 men archers bettered 12 of them on 115 occasions between March and August 1978.

In the Sino-Japanese Archery Friendly Competition of 1979, Meng Fanai bettered the women's 70-metre single-round world record by scoring 321 points. In the same year, 17 national records were broken by eight archers and four teams on 23 occasions.

Sixteen more national records were renewed in 1980 by seven archers and 12 teams on 43 occasions, including 11 men's records on 37 occasions and five women's on six occasions. At the First Asian Cup held in India in February that year, the Chinese women's team carried off five of the six gold medals, four silver and three bronze medals, and the men's team, two bronze medals. At the international tournament held in Romania in May, the Chinese men's team captured the team title, while the women's team placed first in all the six events.

At the Second International Archery Invitational Tournament held in Bucharest in April 1981, Feng Zemin won gold medals for the men's single-round all-round, 90-metre, 50-metre and 60-metre events and a silver medal for the single-round 70-metre event; Hao Shengqi, silver medals for the single-round 90-metre and 50-metre events; Song Shuxian, gold medals for the women's single-round all-round, 70-metre, 60-metre and 50-metre events; and Kong Yaping, silver medal for the women's single-round 60-metre event. The Chinese archery team participated in the world championships for the first time in June 1981 and placed third in the women's total team score, 22 points less than the champion Soviet team, nine points less than the runner-up south Korean team, and 63 points more than the fourth place winner, the U.S.

team. Fu Hong from the Chinese women's team won the 70-metre individual title, and Meng Fanai the 60-metre individual title.

Shooting Shooting, which has a broad popular base in China, is a favourite sport of young people. Up to 1979, more than 10 million people had passed the qualifying test of marksman, and 130,000 shooters had won sportsmen's titles of different classes throughout the whole country. In the 30-plus years since the founding of New China, Chinese men and women shooters have broken national records on more than 600 occasions. Between 1959 when a world record was broken by a Chinese man pistol shooter and May 1981, 19 Chinese shooters broke 16 world records on 34 occasions.

At the Eighth Asian Games in December 1978, the Chinese team garnered eight gold medals and placed first in total team score. At the Third Asian Shooting Championships, Chinese shooters took altogether 13 champion titles, including all the six women's titles.

Chinese sharpshooters achieved remarkable results in 1979. In that year, they surpassed four world records and equalled four, and 24 national records were renewed by 22 shooters and 21 teams on 54 occasions.

More accomplishments were achieved at the national and international competitions of 1980. A men's world record was broken, a women's equalled, and 11 Asian records were bettered. Eight shooters and two teams broke seven national records on 10 occasions. Six of these shooters matched the scores of the first six winners at the 22nd Olympic Games, and 55 shooters matched the level of the first three winners at the 42nd World Championships.

At the national competition of sharpshooters held in

April 1981, Xie Yili's score of 390 points surpassed the running bore mixed-run world record, and Wen Zhifang's score of 592 points equalled the women's small-bore pistol centre-fire world record.

Generally speaking, shooting in China is still behind the advanced world level. This is mainly manifested in Chinese shooters' lack of experience in large-scale international competitions, insufficient mastery of basic skills and lack of consistency in performance. They still have a long way to go in such events as the men's free small-bore rifle and clay pigeon shooting. By comparison, women are doing better than men.

Parachuting New China's first batch of parachutists was trained in 1950. From 1958, when Hao Jianhua and two others broke the women's 1,000-metre day-time team accuracy parachuting world record at the First National Gliding and Parachuting Contests in Beijing, to December 1980, 74 Chinese parachutists bettered 22 world records on 42 occasions.

At the Fourth National Games in 1979, all the national records in the six parachuting events in the competition were broken. 16-year-old Zhang Jianzhong came in first after successively landing on the spot 27 times. His 32 landings on the spot in the individual and team events raised China's national record of individual accuracy to a new level. At the World 4-Man and 8-Man Team Parachuting Championships held in France in August 1979 in which 19 countries participated, the Chinese team won two fourth places. In the same year, four national records were improved by 24 persons and 23 teams on 54 occasions.

China began to attract the attention of world parachuting fans in August 1980 when its men's team placed sixth and its women's team fourth in team total points at the 15th World Parachuting Championships held in Bulgaria. At the National Air-borne Parachuting Contests and the China-Canada-U.S. Parachuting Friendly Contests, both held in November 1980, Chinese parachutists broke one and equalled two world records. In the three-nation contests, the Chinese team captured seven first places, and the U.S. and Canadian teams each took one.

Model Aeroplane Flying The sport of flying model aeroplanes in competition involves knowledge of science and technology. After it started in 1951, model aeroplane flying quickly became a favourite pastime of students after school. Between April 1959, when Wang Gong became the first Chinese to break a world record, and 1965, 32 athletes broke 14 world records on 27 occasions, 45 per cent of the total announced then by the International Aeronautical Federation.

The year 1979 was a peak year for Chinese model aeroplane enthusiasts who bettered eight world records and equalled two. Eleven national records were also bettered by 97 persons on 82 occasions. In the model aeroplane competitions at the Fourth National Games that year, five world records were broken by five persons on five occasions, and one world record was equalled by one person. Bertrand Larcher, Director General of the International Aeronautical Federation, participated in the ceremony in Beijing to award certificates officially approving the world records to the Chinese Aeronautical Association. Three more world records, also approved by the International Aeronautical Federation, were set by four Chinese after the National Games. In October 1979, Chinese aeromodelists took part for the first time in the

World Aeromodel Championships held in Los Angeles, where Gao Qinfei won sixth place in free flight aeroplanes.

At the 1980 World Championships for Tow-Line Controlled Model Aeroplane Flying held in August in Czestochowa, Poland, the Chinese team placed fifth in the F2B tow-line controlled stunt flying. In the same year, two more world records were bettered by two Chinese aeromodelists.

At the Fourth Open Tournament of Radio-Controlled Model Aeroplane Stunt Flying held in Thailand in March 1981, the Chinese team captured the team title, and the Chinese contestant Han Zhongsheng won second place in the individual events.

Model Ships Model ship building, especially popular in China among middle and primary school students, was introduced as a sport in 1954. Since that time, its standard has steadily improved. Eleven national competitions were held between 1958 and 1980, the largest one taking place in 1978 in which over 200 contestants competed in eight events with 181 model ships of their own design. At the Fourth National Games held in 1979, four model ship records were broken by 20 contestants on 64 occasions. At the National Model Ship Contest held in Guangzhou in October 1980, Ge Meng and Su Weibin broke two world records on three occasions. At the contest held in Hangzhou in June 1981, Hu Shenggao, Han-Yongjin, Ge Meng and Chen Liang broke three world records on five occasions.

Mountaineering Nine of the 14 mountains in the world that rise above 8,000 metres are located in or on the border of China. The highest of them all, Mount Qomolangma straddles the Sino-Nepalese border and soars

8,848.13 metres above sea level as the summit of the globe. A mountainous country, China's vast territory is studded with even more mountains of 5,000-7,000 metres in height — all good sites for mountaineering.

When Chinese mountaineers in 1956 scaled the 3,787-metre Mount Taibai in Shaanxi Province to initiate the beginning of modern mountaineering in China, world mountaineering already had a history of more than 170 years.

Following the scaling of Mount Taibai, Chinese mountaineers have since conquered Mount Gongga, the principal peak of the Daxue Mountains; Mount Shule of the Qilian Mountains; Mount Muztagata and Mount Kongur Jiubie of the Kunlun Mountains; the northeast peak of the Nyainqentanglha; the peak of the A'nye-maqen; Mount Tomur, the principal peak of the Tianshan Mountains; and more than 30 peaks of the Karakorum Mountains. They have three times ascended mountains higher than 8,000 metres — twice to the summit of Mount Qomolangma from the northern slope and once to the top of Mount Xixabangma, the last previously unscaled peak above 8,000 metres. They have seven times climbed mountains higher than 7,000 metres and scaled more than 30 peaks above 6,000 metres. So far, 12 Chinese men and women mountaineers have ascended Qomolang-ma, 54 have climbed above 8,500 metres, and 130 have climbed above 8,000 metres.

The Chinese women's mountaineering team went above the 7,500-metre mark in 1959, the second year after the formation of the team, creating a world record for height reached by women climbers at that time. In 1961, they broke their own record.

On May 25, 1960, the Chinese mountaineers Wang

Fuzhou, Gongbu and Qu Yinhua conquered Qomolangma from the northern slope. The same feat was repeated on May 27, 1975 by Phanthog, a woman climber, and eight men climbers, Sodnam Norbu, Lotse, Hou Shengfu, Samdrub, Darphuntso, Kunga Pasang, Tsering Tobgyal and Ngapa Khyen. The ascent was remarkable both in that it involved the first woman to reach the summit from the northern slope and in that a record number of climbers reached the summit of Qomolangma.

5. PHYSICAL EDUCATION AND SCIENTIFIC RESEARCH

Colleges of Physical Education The 11 colleges of physical education in China were all founded after the birth of the People's Republic. The Shanghai Physical Culture Institute founded in 1952, the Beijing and Wuhan physical culture institutes in 1953, and the Xi'an, Chengdu and Shenyang physical culture institutes in 1954 were followed later by physical culture institutes in Tianjin, Guangzhou, Harbin, Shandong and Fujian. These institutes, which offer courses ranging from two to four years, had by 1980 turned out 28,200 graduates (including post graduates). Nearly 1,400 graduated in 1979 and more than 900 in 1980. The 1980 enrolment totalled over 1,900. There are now 9,000 students studying in these institutes under more than 2,100 teachers. Some of the physical culture institutes offer refresher, short-term, correspondence and evening courses. In addition to these institutes, there are the Physical Culture Teachers' College in Beijing and the physical culture departments in 110-plus teachers' colleges in the whole country, where a large number of teachers are trained. A physical culture college of the Chinese People's Liberation Army was founded in 1953. Graduates from this college over the past two decades have become the backbone of physical culture and sports in the armed forces.

Junior Spare-Time Sports Schools The first junior spare-time sports schools were set up in 1955 in Beijing, Shanghai and Tianjin. Later, such schools appeared in all parts of the country. Promising children from primary and secondary schools are enrolled in the sports schools for training after class and on holidays. After an evaluation in 1959, a number of key sports schools were established where the young trainees live, study and train together, spending half the day in study and the other half in training. By 1965, there were more than 1,800 different types of junior spare-time sports schools in the country with a total enrolment of 150,000, who are coached by nearly 3,000 professional instructors. These schools have succeeded in training many first-rate sportsmen and sportswomen.

Work in junior spare-time sports training was strengthened after 1976. In 1978, awards were given to 300 outstanding coaches in spare-time sports training, four of whom also received medals of honour in sports. The State Physical Culture and Sports Commission and the Ministry of Education jointly issued in 1979 new regulations regarding junior spare-time sports schools and compiled new training programmes and teaching materials for 11 sports. According to the overall arrangement made by the State Physical Culture and Sports Commission in 1980, the various provinces, municipalities and autonomous regions reorganized their sports schools to place stress on their specialized sports, laid down or perfected regulations, and improved the quality of instruction. Changes were also made in the way competitions were organized to avoid the tendency of stressing results alone to the neglect of laying a good foundation for the development of talent. The changes emphasized that competitions should benefit young sports enthusiasts in two respects — the building of a good physique and the mastery of basic skills. These measures facilitated the growth of the junior spare-time sports schools. By the end of 1980, ordinary spare-time sports schools had increased to 2,155 with an enrolment of more than 180,000; key spare-time sports schools had increased to 239 with an enrolment of nearly 25,000; more than 9,000 students were receiving training in over 500 key classes; there were 26 physical culture and sports schools with over 5,000 students, and 41 secondary physical culture schools with over 3,000 students. The total enrolment of all the above schools numbered more than 220,000 who were training under 12,000 professional coaches. The courses included track and field, gymnastics, swimming, football, basketball, volleyball, table tennis, badminton, tennis, handball, water polo, diving, speed skating, figure skating, ice hockey, skiing, weightlifting, *wushu*, wrestling, sports acrobatics, cycling, shooting, *xiangqi*, model aeroplanes, *weiqi* (go), baseball, fencing, softball, motorcycling, archery, canoeing, model ships, motorboating, radio transmission and reception, radio engineering and international chess.

The junior spare-time sports schools have played an important role in training a large number of top sportsmen and sportswomen, raising the technical level of sports in China and conducting popular sports activities. Between 1971 and 1979, some 288 trainees in seven sports from the Shichahai Junior Spare-Time Sports School in Beijing joined the best teams in the country. Not a few of them, including Song Xiaobo, a principal player on the national women's basketball team, and Ma Yanhong, world champion on the uneven bars in gymnastics, have won international fame. Sports stars in China like Li Furong (table tennis), Ge Xinai (table tennis), Chen Xiaoxia (diving), Chen Weiqiang (weightlifting), Zou Zhenxian (triple jump), Zheng Dazhen (high jump), Lang Ping (volleyball), Luan Jujie (fencing) and many others have all received training in spare-time sports schools.

Scientific Research in Sports Systematic scientific sports research began with the establishment of a research department in the Beijing Physical Culture Institute. The first specialized organizations — the Beijing Institute of Sports Science and the Beijing Institute of Sports Medicine — both came into existence in 1958. These were followed by research institutes in Shanghai and Heilongjiang and the departments of sports medicine and sports history set up by the Chengdu Physical Culture Institute. By 1980, most provinces and municipalities had set up a sports research institute or department, expanding the ranks of research personnel in the country.

The Institute of Sports Science of the State Physical Culture and Sports Commission (formerly the Beijing Institute of Sports Science) is a general multi-disciplinary research organization composed of research departments of sports training, sports biomechanics, training in ball games, public sports, sports physiology, sports medicine, and information.

A symposium of sports science, the first of its kind, was held in 1956, sponsored by the Beijing Physical Culture Institute, and the First National Conference on Sports

Science and Technology was convened in 1960. In 1964, the State Physical Culture and Sports Commission set up a sports science committee and convened the First National Symposium of Sports Science, which received 321 academic papers recommended by 82 units throughout the country. About 20 per cent of 109 of these papers read at the symposium reached or approached international standards.

In recent years, sports research has made new progress. A national conference was convened by the State Physical Culture and Sports Commission in December 1977 to draw up plans for the development of sports science and technology from 1978 to 1985. The Second National Conference on Sports Science and Technology was held in May 1979 for exchanging experience in sports research and discussing the future tasks and the organizational aspect of research institutions.

To study the morphology of Chinese athletes, the research institute of the State Physical Culture and Sports Commission, the Beijing Physical Culture Institute and some other units made a general survey of 5,175 top sportsmen and sportswomen in 11 sports, including track and field, gymnastics, swimming, weightlifting and ball games. After thirty-three measurements were taken of each athlete, researchers compiled some 200,000 statistical figures to provide fairly comprehensive and complete information about the builds of Chinese sportsmen and sportswomen. This information may serve as a reference in the instruction and training of athletes. Workers in sports medicine also have conducted in-depth research into injuries suffered in sports to determine their causes, including long-term and systematic study of injuries to joints and cartilage which are among the most serious impediments to training. Some of China's achievements in this area have been among the best in the world.

The national symposium of sports science held in December 1980 was a great step forward compared with the one held in 1964. This was shown: 1) In the extended ranks of researchers. For example, 199 units delivered a total of 621 papers, of which 280 were selected and 257 were read at the symposium. 2) In the increased number of disciplines and fields of study. In addition to sports training, sports teaching, sports physiology and sports medicine, there were studies in sports theory and history, tests of physical performance, sports psychology and biomechanics, and sports apparatus and equipment. 3) In the introduction of new methods and means of research. 4) In the marked improvement in the academic standard and practical value of the results of research. 5) In the notable increase in the comprehensive application of the theories and technical means of several disciplines for the joint accomplishment of research tasks. A study of the morphology, physical performance and body structure of young people and children in China, their characteristics and patterns of change and growth has been conducted jointly by the State Physical Culture and Sports Commission, the Ministry of Education and the Ministry of Public Health. Over 1,500 scientists and teachers carried out tests on 180,000 individuals living in 16 provinces and municipalities to collect some 4.4 million useful statistics which are providing basic data for the study of the physique of the Chinese nation. This is an admirable scientific achievement.

But sports science still has a long way to go in China before it can reach world advanced levels. The overall work of sports science has yet to be prefected, and a complete system of sports science has yet to be formed. Research methods are comparatively backward with some new branches of science — cybernetics, information theory and systematology — yet to be applied in sports research. And the gathering and processing of data and information have to be improved to suit the actual needs. Until research in sports science advances quickly enough, training and competition will be carried out for the most part according to conventional methods, hampering the improvement of technical skills. The question of how to strengthen scientific research in sports is now receiving wide attention.

6. SPORTS ORGANIZATIONS, PERSONNEL AND FACILITIES

Sports Organizations The State Physical Culture and Sports Commission of the People's Republic of China is a ministerial government agency, which gives unified guidance to physical culture and sports throughout the country. Local commissions at the provincial, municipal, autonomous regional, prefectural and county levels are responsible for work in their respective localities.

The All-China Sports Federation is a nationwide mass sports organization. Its task is to coordinate with the government to promote sports, publicize and encourage popular sports, organize national competitions, and sponsor and participate in international sports activities. It has branches all over the country.

Affiliated with the All-China Sports Federation are associations of individual sports, which, as mass sports organizations, have the following tasks: to publicize and promote their respective sports, organize competitions, study the methods of training and raise skills. There are national and local associations, such as the Football Association of the People's Republic of China and the Football Association of Shanghai. The national associations establish relations with their counterparts in other countries for international competitions and other activities. There are at present more than 30 national associations, devoted respectively to track and field, swimming, gymnastics, sports acrobatics, basketball, volleyball, football, table tennis, badminton, tennis, handball, baseball and softball, weightlifting, cycling, wrestling, fencing, *weiqi* (go), *xiangqi* (Chinese chess), archery, shooting, radio transmission and reception, model aeroplanes, model ships, mountaineering, winter sports, *wushu* (martial arts), etc.

The Chinese Olympic Committee is a national sports organization with the duties of promoting sports and the Olympic games. As the sole organization representing the Olympic Movement in China, it sends delegations to the Olympic Games and the Winter Olympic Games and maintains relations with the International Olympic Committee and the Olympic Committees of various countries.

The departments of education, the Communist Youth League and trade unions in China have their own sports organizations to take charge of work in sports in their own departments. The Ministry of Education, for example, has a physical culture department. The local bureaus of education also have physical culture departments of their own. Teaching and research sections of physical culture are to be found in all universities and colleges.

Sports Stars of 1979 A popularity poll to pick 10 top sports stars of 1979 was jointly sponsored by the

Central People's Broadcasting Station, *Sports News* and two other organizations. The winners were:

Chen Xiaoxia — A new diving star, the 17-year-old girl from Guangdong dethroned the Soviet Union's world champion Irina Kalinina and captured the 10-metre platform title at the 10th Universiad in September 1979. She achieved distinction with a series of extremely difficult movements, graceful performances, rapid twists and turns and flawless entries into the water.

Chen Weiqiang — The 21-year-old weightlifter is also from Guangdong Province. In 1979, he twice broke the 56 kg-class clean and jerk world record by lifting 151.5 kg and then 153 kg. In 1977 and 1978, he toppled the world youth record on five occasions.

Ge Xinai — This 26-year-old table tennis player from Henan captured the title of the women's singles and, in cooperation with her teammates, won the mixed doubles and women's team event titles at the 35th World Table Tennis Championships in 1979.

Wu Shude — Born in Nanning, Guangxi Zhuang Autonomous Region, this 20-year-old weightlifter is a new world champion. He bettered the 52 kg-class world youth records of snatch and in total points on five occasions in 1979, and won the 52 kg-class snatch title at the World Weightlifting Championships held in Greece in November that year.

Rong Zhihang — A native of Guangdong Province, the 31-year-old veteran football player is known for his skilful dribbling, fast breaking play and good sportsmanship, which people praise as the "Zhihang Style". He has been a high scorer in many international matches.

Nie Weiping — At 27, this *weiqi* (go) player from Heilongjiang Province won several national titles and repeatedly outplayed Japanese 9th-grade ace players between 1973 and 1979. Japanese go players call him "Nie the Whirlwind".

Luan Jujie — The 21-year-old woman foil fencer from Nanjing, Jiangsu Province, defeated eight European fencers and won a silver medal at the 29th World Junior Fencing Championships in 1978, thus breaking the monopoly by the Europeans in fencing. She was praised as the "No. 1 woman fencer of Asia" after winning the women's foil championship at the Eighth Asian Games.

Zou Zhenxian — This 24-year-old Asian record holder in triple jump is from Dalian, Liaoning Province. He again broke the Asian record in June 1979 with a jump of 17.02 metres, ranking himself seventh among the world's triple jumpers of the time.

Song Xiaobo — The 21-year-old forward of the Beijing Women's Basketball Team has been repeatedly named a best player in national and international competitions. She is 1.82 metres tall.

Wu Xinshui — Though already 35 and only 1.78 metres tall, he is the "soul" of the August 1st Men's Basketball Team. He scored 25 individual points in the team's first match against an American team in 1979.

Sports Stars of 1980 More than 170,000 voted in the poll to select 10 top sports stars of 1980 sponsored by 10 units of the mass media in Beijing. The winners were:

Chen Xiaoxia — Winner of the greatest number of votes as last year, she captured the gold medal in the women's platform diving event in the Martini International Diving Competition held in November 1980, outscoring many world-famous divers by a distinct margin.

Lang Ping — The 20-year-old from Beijing is the No. 1 spiker on the national women's volleyball team. She is

1.84 metres tall and her jump reaches as high as 3.17 metres. Her powerful spikes won many points for her team in the matches against the Japanese, American and other strong teams in 1980. She was named the "Best Spiker" in the Bremen international tournament in West Germany.

Liang Weifen — The 18-year-old swimmer was born in a boat family in Guangdong Province. She won seven gold medals at the international swimming contest held in July 1980 in Yugoslavia. In August that year, she defeated the well-known American swimmer Tracy Caulkins in Beijing, and later captured the title in the women's 100-metre breaststroke at the Hawaii invitational in 1:12.84, which is Asia's best time.

Guo Yaohua — Born in Xiamen, Fujian Province, the 24-year-old table tennis player was twice runner-up in world table tennis championships. He won the men's singles title at the first world cup in 1980.

Wu Shude — A repeat poll winner, Wu broke the 52 kg-class world record with a snatch of 112 kg in the 1980 National Weightlifting Championships and placed second in total points for the 56 kg-class in the International Weightlifting Tournament held in Honolulu.

Rong Zhihang — Another second-time winner, Rong gave the best of himself and played a leader's role in carrying the Chinese football team through to victory in the World Cup Asian-Oceanian Zone Group 4 Qualifying Tournament held in Hongkong in January 1981 and was honoured as the Best Striker there.

Li Yuejiu — A gymnast of 23 from Liaoning Province, Li is noted for his perseverance and creativeness in performing dangerous and highly difficult movements. He won the floor exercise event at the Hartford tournament in 1980 and came in first on the parallel bars and second in the floor exercise at the World Cup '80 held in Canada.

Li Cuiling — The 20-year-old gymnast from Inner Mongolia was the winner of the individual all-round title at the 1980 Hartford tournament where she also played a part in winning the team title for the Chinese women's team. At the Nagoya international tournament held in November, she placed first in the individual all-round event and on the vaulting horse and the balance beam.

Han Jian — Hailing from Shenyang in Liaoning Province, this 24-year-old Chinese shuttler was the winner of the men's singles at the World Cup badminton competitions held in 1979. He created an international sports sensation when he defeated the Indonesian "badminton king" Liem Swie King at the China-Indonesia duel that took place in February 1980.

Zou Zhenxian — Also elected in 1979, he won the triple jump title at the Liberty Bell Track and Field Classic held in Philadelphia in July 1980 and came in first again at the Beijing International Invitational in September. His unique method of taking off by swinging up both of his arms has been described as the "Zou Style".

Sports Stars of 1981 More than 250,000 votes were turned in during the nationwide poll conducted by 18 mass media organizations in Beijing to select the 10 top sports stars of 1981. The winners were:

Sun Jinfang — The 27-year-old captain of the Chinese women's volleyball team was the key organizer on court of her team's powerful offence. By fostering a dauntless spirit to fight on, she steered her team to victory at the 1981 Third World Cup women's volleyball championship held in Japan where she was awarded three prizes — Best Athlete, Fine Athlete and Setter.

Lang Ping — This 21-year-old girl from Beijing is the famous "iron hammer" of the Chinese women's volleyball team and one of the three best spikers in the world. She played a prominent part in her team's winning the championship title at the Third World Cup competition and was awarded the Fine Athlete prize. She was named one of the 10 top sports stars in 1980.

Chen Xiaoxia — This young Guangdong woman has been a gold medalist in all the important international diving competitions since 1978. She won the top honour at the World Cup diving competition in June 1981 and captured the gold medal with unusually high points in the platform diving competition at the Universiad in July. She is a third-time winner in the rating for 10 Best Athletes.

Guo Yaohua — Runner-up in the men's singles event at the 34th and 35th World Table Tennis Championships, Guo succeeded in capturing the title in the same event at the 36th World Championships in 1981. He was re-elected as one of the 10 Best Athletes following his election in 1980.

Rong Zhihang — This veteran is the "soul" of the Chinese football team. For his outstanding performance as a play-maker in the 1981 World Cup Asian-Oceanian Zone finals, he was chosen for the third time in the Best Athletes election.

Li Yuejiu — A "veteran" gymnast, Li has developed many new and highly difficult stunts rarely seen in world gymnastics. He won the gold medal in the floor exercise at the 21st World Gymnastics Championships in 1981 and was re-elected a Best Athlete after 1980.

Zou Zhenxian — This world-known triple jumper broke three Asian records and a Universiad record in 1981. He was the runner-up at the Third World Cup track and field competition, and his best record of 17.34 metres ranked him the third best in the world in 1981. He is also a three-time winner in the 10 Best Athletes election.

Tong Ling — A 19-year-old from Zigong, Sichuan Province, she was the women's singles champion at the 36th World Table Tennis Championships in 1981.

Wu Shude — At the 1981 Asian Weightlifting Championships, he broke the 56 kg-class snatch world record by lifting 126.5 kilogrammes. Known as "the man who breaks world records every year", Wu was elected a Best Athlete for the third time in 1981.

Li Xiaoping — The 19-year-old new gymnastics star has been praised as a "wonder horse-rider" in international competitions. He captured the title on the pommel horse at the 21st World Gymnastics Championships in 1981 by scoring a full 10 points.

Titles of Sportsmen In April 1956, the State Physical Culture and Sports Commission promulgated the draft Regulations for Conferring Sportsmen's Titles of the People's Republic of China and the standards for winning titles of different classes. Revised in 1958 and then in 1963, these regulations specify titles of five classes: Master of Sports, First-Class Sportsman, Second-Class Sportsman, Third-Class Sportsman and Junior Sportsman. By the end of 1965, more than 10.713 million sportsmen had qualified for one or another of these titles. Among them, 3,338 had won the Master of Sports title.

In July 1978, the State Physical Culture and Sports Commission proclaimed the Technical Grading System of Sportsmen (Revised Draft) for trial implementation. The system stipulates that any sportsman who meets the required qualifications and standards is conferred with a corresponding title. In 1978 and 1979, more than 32,000 sportsmen became title holders and 463 of them were awarded the title of Master of Sports by the State Physical Culture and Sports Commission. Over 47,200 more sportsmen joined the ranks of the title holders in 1980, among them 1,147 Masters of Sports.

Titles of Coaches The State Physical Culture and Sports Commission promulgated a Grading System of Coaches in 1958 and had it revised in 1963. But the system was not put into effect before 1966. A new Technical Grading System of Coaches (Draft) was issued in June 1979, conferring titles of five different classes on sports coaches who meet the required qualifications. These are National Coach, First-Class Coach, Second-Class Coach, Third-Class Coach and Assistant Coach. By the end of 1980, 846 coaches, among them 213 National Coaches, had been granted titles.

Titles of Judges The State Physical Culture and Sports Commission promulgated the Draft Regulations for the Grading System of Judges of the People's Republic of China in April 1956 and revised it in 1958 and 1963. According to the regulations, there were four classes of judges: National Judge, and First-Class, Second-Class and Third-Class Judges. Sports judges who meet the qualifications are given appropriate titles. By the end of 1965, there were more than 1.41 million judges who had acquired a title, 803 of whom that of National Judge.

The revised Grading System of Judges was promulgated by the State Physical Culture and Sports Commission in June 1978. Between 1978 and 1979, China had more than 38,900 judges, among them 1,107 National Judges. More than 43,400 judges, including 435 National Judges, were given titles of different classes in 1980.

Between 1974 and 1980, 95 Chinese were approved as International Judges in nine sports by the relevant international organizations of individual sports.

Sports Facilities In the past three decades or more, the central and local governments have built a large number of stadiums, gymnasiums, indoor and outdoor swimming pools, shooting ranges, training halls and other sports facilities. By the end of 1980, there were 160-plus stadiums in the whole country with fixed stands (including 40 with a seating capacity for 25,000 or more spectators), 14 times as many as in 1949; and 130 gymnasiums of all types (including more than 30 with a seating capacity of 4,000), 11 times as many as in 1949. There were 1,390 swimming pools, over 13 times more than in 1949, and 2,200-plus lighted ball courts with fixed stands in addition to large numbers of less well-equipped facilities including the nearly 600 indoor and outdoor facilities for basketball, volleyball, football, table tennis, badminton, gymnastics, weightlifting, swimming, shooting and other sports built in 1979 and 1980. Many organizations have their own courts and sports grounds.

The Beijing Gymnasium built in 1955, has a competition hall with 6,000 seats, a swimming hall with 2,000 seats and a practice hall. The Beijing Workers' Stadium, completed in 1959 on the 10th anniversary of the founding of New China, is the largest all-purpose stadium in China today, its buildings covering a floor space of 80,000 square metres. Its central stadium with a capacity for 80,000 spectators is surrounded by basketball, volleyball and tennis courts, football fields and indoor and outdoor swimming pools. The Beijing Workers' Gymnasium with seats for 15,000 spectators was built in 1961. Its round dome is suspended by steel cables, and its competition hall, where the 26th World Table Tennis Championships were held, is 40 metres in diameter.

The Capital Gymnasium in Beijing is also one of the largest in China. Built in 1968, it is 122 metres long, 107 metres wide and 28 metres high, with seats for 18,000 spectators. Its 88-by-40-metre competition court is ideal for basketball, volleyball, table tennis and badminton matches and gymnastic competitions. With the floor removed, the court can be turned into an ice rink by artificial refrigeration for ice hockey matches or figure skating competitions. The gymnasium is air-conditioned and equipped with a refrigerating system and other modern installations, including radio and television relay, radio facsimile, lighting, timing and communication facilities.

All told, there are more than 30 public stadiums, gymnasiums and sports fields in Beijing in frequent use by sports fans. The principal stadiums and gymnasiums cover a total floor space of over 200,000 square metres and have an aggregate capacity for 210,000 spectators. Other facilities include a parachuting tower, water sports club, motorcycling track, cycling track, baseball and softball courts and indoor air-rifle ranges.

The Shanghai Gymnasium was built in 1975 and is equipped with modern facilities. Its buildings, including the competition hall, practice hall, hostel and a chamber housing the refrigerating apparatus, cover a total floor space of 47,000 square metres. Its circular competition hall is 110 metres in diameter and can hold 18,000 spectators.

An outdoor mechanically refrigerated speed-skating rink, one of the best equipped ice skating training centres in China, was built in Changchun in 1978.

The construction of large indoor stadiums in recent years in the cities of Beijing, Shanghai, Nanjing, Shenyang, Jinan, Fuzhou and Hohhot has been accompanied by the mushrooming of smaller ones with a seating capacity of 4,000 or so in some medium cities, including Hengyang, Xiangtan and Zhuzhou in Hunan Province, Wuxi, Zhenjiang and Suzhou in Jiangsu Province, Liuzhou in Guangxi Zhuang Autonomous Region; and Shaoguan in Guangdong Province.

7. INTERNATIONAL CONTACTS

Friendly Exchanges Sports is a "bridge" of friendship between the people of different countries. In the last 30 years or more, most of the people in the international sports world have been friendly to the Chinese people. Despite some unpleasant disruptions and interferences, China's sports organizations have established ever more extensive and closer contacts with those of other countries and international sports organizations.

In 1978, reciprocal visits were exchanged between China and 92 other countries and regions, involving over 340 sports delegations and teams and more than 5,600 persons. In 1979, there were 450 such visits by 5,200 persons between China and 92 other countries and regions. In 1980, China sent more than 3,300 persons in 220 delegations or teams to 68 countries and regions from which came more than 2,500 visitors in 140 delegations or teams.

Statistics reveal that in the 31 years between 1949

and 1980, China exchanged visits with over 100 countries and regions in the world, involving nearly 60,000 persons in 4,000 groups.

In international competitions, China adheres to the principle of "friendship first, competition second" and the principle of equality and mutual respect without regard to the size of countries. Through extensive international competitions and sports exchanges, the Chinese people have strengthened their unity with the people of other countries, acquainted themselves with their advanced experience and thus promoted the growth of sports in China.

World and Asian Sports Organizations of Which China Is a Member

Table 1

	Year of Founding	*Year of Joining or Resumption of China's Membership*
Comité Internationale Olimpique (CIO)	1894	1922, 1958,* 1979**
International Amateur Athletic Federation (IAAF)	1912	1928, 1958,* 1978**
Fédération Internationale des Sociétés d'Aviron (FISA)	1892	1973
Fédération Internationale de Basketball Amateur (FIBA)	1932	1936, 1958,* 1974**

* Year of withdrawal.
** Year of resumption of membership.

Fédération Internationale de Canoë (FIC)	1924	1974
Fédération Internationale Amateur de Cyclisme (FIAC)	1900	1939, 1958,* 1979**
Fédération Internationale d'Escrime (FIE)	1913	1974
Fédération Internationale de Football Association (FIFA)	1904	1931, 1958,* 1979**
Fédération Internationale de Gymnastique (FIG)	1881	1956, 1964,* 1978**
International Weightlifting Federation (IWF)	1920	1936, 1958,* 1974**
International Handball Federation (IHF)	1946	1979
Fédération Internationale de Hockey (FIH)	1924	1980
International Ice Hockey Federation (IIHF)	1908	1957
Fédération Internationale de Lutte Amateur (FILA)	1911	1936, 1958,* 1974**
Fédération Internationale de Natation Amateur (FINA)	1908	1954, 1958,* 1980**
International Skating Union (ISU)	1892	1956
Fédération Internationale de Ski (FIS)	1924	1981
Union Internationale de Tir (UIT)	1905	1954, 1958,* 1979**

Fédération Internationale de Tir à l'Arc (FITA)	1931	1967, 1971,* 1981**
Fédération Internationale de Volley-Ball (FIVB)	1947	1952, 1970,* 1974**
Fédération Aeronautique Internationale (FAI)	1905	1978
International Federation of Sports Acrobatics (IFSA)	1973	1979
World Badminton Federation (WBF)	1978	1978
International Badminton Federation (IBF)	1939	1981 (WBF and IBF amalgamated)
World Bridge Federation (WBF)	1958	1980
Fédération Internationale des Echecs (FIDE)	1924	1966, 1970,* 1975**
Fédération Internationale Motocycliste (FIM)	1904	1979
Union Internationale Motonautique (UIM)	1922	1980
World Organization for Modelshipbuilding and Modelshipsport (NAVIGA)	1959	1980
Fédération Internationale de Rollers Skating (FIRS)	1924	1980
International Softball Federation (ISF)	1952	1979

International Table Tennis Federation (ITTF)	1926	1953
Comité Intergourvernemental pour l'Education Physique et le Sport (CIEPSUNESCO)	1958	1978
International Assembly of National Confederations of Sport (IANCS)	1981	1981
International Association for Sports Information (IASI)	1960	1981
Fédération Internationale de Medicine Sportive (FIMS)	1928	1980
Conseil International du Sport Militaire (CISM)	1948	1979
Association Internationale de la Presse Sportive (AIPS)	1924	1979
Fédération Internationale du Sport Scolalre (ISF)	1972	1973
Fédération Internationale du Sport Universitaire (FISU)	1949	1975

Table 2

	Year of Joining
Asian Table Tennis Union (ATTU)	1972
Asian Games Federation (AGF)	1973
Asian Football Confederation (AFC)	1974
Asian Cycling Federation (ACF)	1974
Asian Weightlifting Federation (AWF)	1974
Asian Gymnastic Confederation (AGC)	1974
Asian Wrestling Committee (AWC)	1974
Fencing Confederation of Asia (FCA)	1974
Asian Badminton Confederation (ABC)	1974
Asian Shooting Confederation (ASC)	1974
Asian Basketball Confederation (ABC)	1975
Asian Volleyball Confederation (AVC)	1975

Asian Handball Federation (AHF)	1976
Asian Amateur Swimming Federation (AASF)	1978
Asian Archery Federation (AAF)	1978
Asian Amateur Athletic Association (AAAA)	1978
Asian Equestrian Federation (AEF)	1978
Asian (Chinese) Chess Federation	1978
Asian Sports Journalists Union (ASJU)	1978

The Chinese Olympic Committee's Relations with the International Olympic Committee The International Olympic Committee recognized China's national sports organization as early as 1922. Three Chinese, including Dong Shouyi, have successively been on the IOC. Old China sent its team to compete in the Olympic Games three times, in 1932, 1936 and 1948, but only Fu Baolu entered pole-vault finals at the 11th Olympic Games of 1936.

After the founding of the People's Republic of China in 1949, the Chinese Olympic Committee was reorganized. The All-China Sports Federation and Dong Shouyi, member of the International Olympic Committee, sent a telegram to the IOC in December 1951, informing it that China intended to participate in the 15th Olympic Games to be held in Helsinki in 1952. As a result of the obstructions, delays and difficulties created by a couple of leading IOC members at the time, a resolution for extending invitation to the Chinese athletes to participate in the 15th Olympic Games was passed by a 32-20 vote only at the 47th session of the IOC two days before the opening of the Olympic Games. When the delegation sent by the Chinese Olympic Committee and composed of 40 athletes (a basketball, a football and a swimming team) arrived in Helsinki, the competitions were already drawing to a close. The Chinese athletes held a ceremony for hoisting the flag of the People's Republic of China, participated in the swimming contest, made friends with athletes of other countries and attended the closing ceremony.

At its 49th plenary session held in Athens in May 1954, the IOC officially recognized the Chinese Olympic Committee by a 32-21 vote. But without being discussed at any IOC meeting, Taiwan's Chinese Amateur Athletic Federation was illegitimately listed among the national Olympic Committees recognized by the IOC, thus creating "two China's" in an international sports organization. The Chinese Olympic Committee discussed this with the IOC many times and lodged repeated protests, to no avail. China had already formed an athletic delegation and made all preparations to take part in the 16th Olympic Games to be held in Melbourne in 1956. But in protest against the IOC's disregard of the Chinese people's legitimate right, China indignantly decided to boycott the Olympic Games, and on August 19, 1958, the Chinese Olympic

Committee announced that it would sever its relations with the IOC.

In April 1975, the Chinese Olympic Committee applied to the IOC demanding the restoration of its right as the sole representative of China in the Olympic Movement.

In March 1979, the IOC Executive Board proposed that the representatives of the Chinese Olympic Committee and the Olympic Committee at Taibei come to a meeting in Lucerne, Switzerland, to be presided over by Lord Killanin. Although China agreed to the proposal, the meeting did not materialize on account of Taiwan's refusal to attend.

The IOC Executive Board met on October 25, 1979 in Nagoya, Japan, and passed a resolution to the effect that the Olympic Committee of the People's Republic of China, by the name of "the Chinese Olympic Committee", is the national Olympic Committee of China, whose flag and anthem are those of the People's Republic of China; and that the Olympic Committee based in Taibei is to stay on the IOC as a regional organization of China under the name of "the Chinese Taibei Olympic Committee", whose flag, anthem and emblem are to be other than those used at present and must be approved by the Executive Board of the IOC. The resolution embodied the principle of one China, was in keeping with the Charter of the international Olympics and took into consideration the actual situation of China's Taiwan area so that all Chinese athletes on China's mainland and in the Taiwan area can participate in the Olympic Games. The resolution was submitted to all IOC members for approval by postal vote. The result of 62 in favour of the resolution and 17 against was announced on November 26. The Chinese

Olympic Committee thus entered into a new stage in its relations with the IOC.

Zhong Shitong, President of the Chinese Olympic Committee, announced at a press conference attended by Chinese and foreign correspondents in Beijing on November 27, 1979 that China had decided to send sports delegations to take part in the competitions of the 13th Winter Olympic Games to be held in Lake Placid, U.S.A, in February 1980, and to take part in the qualifying rounds and competitions of 15 sports, including track and field, swimming and gymnastics, of the 22nd Olympic Games to be held in Moscow in July 1980. On the same day, he wrote a letter to Mr. Shen Chia-ming, Chairman of the Chinese Taibei Olympic Committee, proposing that sports exchanges between the two sides should be realized at an early date. Zhong Shitong solemnly declared that China would like to see that international federations of individual sports follow the example of the IOC resolution in solving the question of providing athletes of all sports in China's Taiwan area with an opportunity to take part in international competitions.

A Chinese sports delegation was present at the 13th Winter Olympic Games where Chinese athletes competed in speed skating, figure skating, skiing and the biathlon. At a plenary session on April 24, 1980, the Chinese Olympic Committee decided to send no sportsmen to the 22nd Olympic Games in Moscow so long as Soviet authorities refused to respect the noble ideals of the Olympic Movement and to withdraw all the Soviet troops from Afghanistan by May 24. The Chinese Olympic Committee would yet send sportsmen to the pre-Olympic trials held outside the Soviet Union. As events later developed, the Olympic

Games in Moscow were boycotted by China and nearly 60 other member countries.

Peaks Open to Foreign Mountaineers Nine of the many high mountains and lofty peaks which abound in China's Tibet, Xinjiang, Sichuan and Qinghai have been open to foreigners since 1980. Mountaineering organizations may submit their applications along with a fee to the Chinese Mountaineering Association which has already received over 100 such requests from scores of countries for permission to scale Chinese mountains.

The nine peaks are: Mount Qomolangma (on the Sino-Nepalese border, 8,848 metres above sea level), Mount Xixabangma (Tibet, 8,012 metres), Mount Kongur (Xinjiang, 7,719 metres), Mount Kongur Jiubie (Xinjiang, 7,595 metres), Mount Gongga (Sichuan, 7,556 metres), Mount Muztagata (Xinjiang, 7,546 metres), Mount A'nyemaqen (Qinghai, 6,282 metres), Mount Bogda (Xinjiang, 5,445 metres), and Mount Siguniang (Sichuan, 6,250 metres).

In 1980, 228 mountaineers in 40 groups from 11 countries came to the nine peaks in China to engage in mountaineering, surveying and tourist activities. Over 50 more delegations were in China for negotiations and signing of mountaineering or mountaineering-tourist agreements.

China Sports Service Founded in Beijing in October 1979, the China Sports Service oversees and organizes China's external commercial activities in sports. In conformity with the principles of equality and mutual benefit, it has established friendly contact and promoted business relations with many sports, economic and trade, advertising and travel circles in other parts of the world. Its scope of business includes: tendering rights for TV or film coverage of domestic or international sports competitions in China; putting up advertisements for foreign commercial establishments in the stadiums or gymnasiums in China; purchasing clothing and equipment for Chinese sports teams from foreign firms; making arrangements for Chinese sports teams to go abroad and foreign teams to come to China for exhibitions or competitions on a commercial basis; receiving visitors coming to China at their own expenses for sports competitions and sightseeing or for training in table tennis, *wushu*, *taijiquan* and other sports; and selling commemorative sports coins to foreign countries.

Chapter Two

MEDICINE AND PUBLIC HEALTH

1. HISTORICAL RETROSPECT

(1) TRADITIONAL CHINESE MEDICINE AND PHARMACOLOGY

A rich treasure-house created by ancient Chinese people in their long years of struggle against disease, traditional Chinese medicine and pharmacology forms an independent school within the healing arts. It has made outstanding achievements over its 2,000-year history during which it has improved continuously to remain widely practised today. It incorporates the *yin* (negative) and *yang* (positive) theory and the theory of the five elements (metal, wood, water, fire and earth), both containing naive dialectical ideas of ancient China. The former theory holds that everything has a *yin* and a *yang* side the struggle and interaction between which is the source of the ceaseless emergence and change of all things in the universe. The latter theory believes that things in the universe are composed of the five indispensable elements of daily life, which move and change constantly to mutually promote and restrain each other.

Beyond theory, the physiological and pathological branches of traditional Chinese medicine focus on the internal organs, main and collateral "channels", "vital energy" ("*qi*") and blood, excretions and discharges. Diagnoses are made within a complete observational system in which the nature of a patient's disease is determined by the "four methods of diagnosis" — observing the overall way the patient looks, listening to the voice and observing any odour, asking questions, and feeling the patient's pulse. Treatment then proceeds to balance the "eight principal syndromes" — *yin* and *yang*, exterior and interior, cold and heat, underactivity and overactivity.

According to traditional Chinese pharmacology, the properties of drugs are differentiated by their "four characteristics" (cold, cool, warm and hot) and their "five tastes" (hot, bitter, salty, sour and sweet).

Other Chinese therapies include acupuncture and moxibustion, which involve the study of "channels" and "points" on the human body, and the methods of treatment by massage, *qigong* (breathing exercises) and *daoyin* (physical exercises).

Traditional Chinese medicine and pharmacology embodies a great many valuable ideas and views which have been proved through practice. One of the most important is that, instead of treating only the symptoms, traditional Chinese medicine takes into consideration every aspect of a patient's condition to form a unified idea of it under the theories of *yin* and *yang* and the five elements before deciding on its treatment. For example, in the case of a disease requiring surgery, Chinese medicine is concerned with the general physiological changes which may have brought about the condition and — beyond operating or applying some form of therapy — seeks to improve the patient's ability to resist the disease. Preventive medicine — so highly acclaimed by people today — has always been stressed in traditional Chinese medicine. Included in its preventive measures are giving early treatment and developing immunities, or "combating evil with evil".

The particular approaches of traditional Chinese medicine and pharmacology have made important contributions to health protection and the development of medicine and pharmacology. Acupuncture and moxibustion treatment, for example, is a unique Chinese method proved remarkably effective in curing many kinds of ailments. Among its merits are its wide scope of application in curing and preventing internal, surgical, gynaecologic and paediatric diseases and diseases of the five sense organs (ear, eye, lip, nose and tongue); its quick and notable curative effect; its easy applicability at a low cost; and its producing little or no side effects.

Treating diseases by acupuncture and moxibustion involves pricking with a needle or cauterizing, with a burning moxa stick, selected points of the human body based on the Chinese medical theory of main and collateral "channels". This method is not only widely applied in China, but is popular in many other countries. It found its way to Korea in the 6th century and then to Japan and Southeast and Central Asia. It became known to Europe in the 17th century.

The experience of traditional doctors in understanding, observing, analysing and treating disease has been handed down mainly through medical literature. According to an incomplete count, there are about 8,000 pieces of such literature extant today, most of them dealing with clinical medicine.

Canon of Medicine (Nei Jing), *Treatise on Febrile and Other Diseases (Shang Han Za Bing Lun)* and *Shen Nong's Materia Medica (Shen Nong Ben Cao Jing)* are three representative early medical works written before the third century B.C. *Canon of Medicine*, the earliest existing Chinese medical masterpiece, was completed during the Warring States Period (475-221 B.C.) and consists of 18 volumes and 162 chapters. It laid the theoretical base of Chinese medicine by giving fairly scientific explanations of the physiological functions of the human body, symptoms of diseases and the principles of diagnosis and treatment. The other two books were written in the Eastern Han Dynasty (A.D. 25-220). *Treatise on Febrile and Other Diseases* deals mainly with the dialectical method of diagnosis, methods of treatment and prescriptions, while *Shen Nong's Materia Medica*, the earliest extant work of pharmacology listing 365 drugs laid the groundwork for Chinese pharmacology.

A large number of medical and pharmacological works appeared after the Han Dynasty. The 10-volume *Classic on Pulse* (*Mai Ming*) compiled by Wang Shuhe in the third century describes in detail 24 different patterns of pulse beats and their diagnostic significance. As China's earliest extant book on the subject, it posited the basic theories behind diagnosis by feeling the pulse. *A Classic of Acupuncture and Moxibustion (Zhen Jiu Jia Yi Jing)* written by Huangfu Mi is the earliest extant book of its kind. It is still considered a must for practitioners of acupuncture and moxibustion today. In the seventh century, Su Jing and his colleagues compiled *Revised Materia Medica* (*Xin Xiu Ben Cao*). This great work of 54 volumes lists 844 medicines and was the first pharmacological book approved by the government and the earliest pharmacopoeia in the world. *Ten Thousand Golden Formulas (Qian Jin Yao Fang)* and *Ten Thousand Golden Supplementary Formulas* (*Qian Jin Yi Fang*), compiled by the famous physician Sun Simiao and each comprising 30 volumes, were a summing-up of the achievements in Chinese medicine and pharmacology before the seventh century. The two books treat in great detail the diagnosis, treatment and prevention of diseases, particularly in gynaecology and paediatrics. *Manual of Forensic Medicine (Xi Yuan Lu)* written by Song Ci in 1247 is the world's earliest systematic work on this branch of medicine. Li Shizhen, a great Ming Dynasty medical scientist of the 16th century, compiled the 52-volume *Compendium of Materia Medica* (*Ben Cao Gang Mu*), which contains descriptions of 1,892 medicinal materials and over 11,000 prescriptions. This encyclopaedia summed up the knowledge and experience of Chinese pharmacology over the preceding 2,000 years. Translated wholly or partly into English, French, German, Japanese, Latin, Korean and some other languages, it has won wide recognition both in China and abroad over the past 400 years.

(2) MEDICINE AND PHARMACOLOGY IN MODERN CHINA

After the Opium War of 1840, as China was gradually reduced to a semi-feudal and semi-colonial status, Western medicine and pharmacology began to be introduced into China on an extensive scale. Before 1840, there were already a number of hospitals set up in Guangdong, Shanghai and other places by missionaries and businessmen from Britain, the United States and other countries. The number of hospitals and medical colleges and schools run by foreign missionaries increased substantially after the war. From 1828 to 1949, such hospitals increased to 340. Beginning with the medical school founded in

Guangzhou by the British Medical Missionary Society in 1866, the number of medical colleges and schools run by foreign missionaries increased to 20 by 1916. The Qing government soon followed suit and established the Beiyang Medical College in Tianjin and the Capital Medical College in Beijing. After the Revolution of 1911 that overthrew the Qing Dynasty (1644-1911), the medical colleges and schools set up in a few cities by the successive governments were all modelled on Western counterparts.

The introduction of Western medicine and pharmacology into China brought new knowledge to promote medical and public health work in the country, but it also gave rise to a tendency to negate China's traditional medicine and pharmacology. The Kuomintang government adopted a resolution in 1929 banning the practice of traditional medicine, which aroused indignation and protests by Chinese medical practitioners throughout the country. This policy failed because, deeply rooted among the people, traditional Chinese medicine and pharmacology had proved its efficacy in curing diseases and preserving health and could by no means be replaced by the Western.

Under the political corruption and economic depression during the Kuomintang rule, medical and health services fell into a deplorable state. In 1949, six of the 22 provinces in the whole country did not even have a governmental department to look after such services. For a country the size of China, there were only 3,670 medical institutions (including 2,600 hospitals) with 505,040 medical technical personnel and 80,000 beds. Two-thirds of these institutions were run by the government. Most of the hospitals were poorly equipped, charged high fees and were concentrated in the major cities. There was an acute shortage of doctors, medicine and medical facilities in the vast countryside. From 1928 to 1947, only 9,499 graduated from medical colleges. The manufacture of Western medicines and medical equipment was also in a backward state. Most of the pharmaceutical factories had to rely on imported materials, which amounted to 7,650 tons in 1946-47. Economic poverty and lack of doctors, medicine and medical facilities led to a general deterioration of the health of the people, prevalence of disease and a rise in the mortality rate. Between 1910 and 1947, plague broke out three times in northeast China, with a death toll of over 100,000. During 50 pre-liberation years, Shanghai had 12 outbreaks of cholera. In the old China, venereal diseases and tuberculosis were common. There was a high incidence of smallpox, typhoid, malaria, leprosy, hookworm disease, puerperal fever and tetanus in the newborn. The national mortality rate before liberation was 25 per thousand and the infant mortality rate 200 per thousand. The average life expectancy of a Chinese was 35 years.

2. MEDICAL AND HEALTH SERVICES IN NEW CHINA

The founding of New China in 1949 opened broad vistas for the development of medical and health services. The People's Government showed a real concern for the health of the people and put forward, early in the post-liberation years, the four principles in health work: To be geared to the needs of the workers, peasants and soldiers; putting prevention first; uniting doctors of both traditional and Western medicine; and combining health work with mass movement. These principles clearly defined the nature of the socialist medical and health services and pointed out their direction: to serve the broad masses of the people and protect their health. A fundamental change took place in health work as the People's Government built and set up a large number of medical and health institutions, trained a great number of medical and health personnel and vigorously launched a mass Patriotic Health Campaign. Many infectious diseases which seriously jeopardized the people's health, such as plague, smallpox, venereal disease, kala-azar, relapsing fever and typhus, have been completely or basically wiped out. Snail fever (schistosomiasis) has been basically eliminated in many provinces and cities, and two-thirds of the over 10 million sufferers have been fully cured. More than 30 million people suffered from malaria before liberation. The number has been reduced to about 3.3 million today, and the rate of malaria occurrence in 862 counties and cities has dropped to below 0.5 per thousand. Many endemic diseases, including Keshan disease and Kaschin-Beck disease, have been more or less placed under control, while the incidence of acute infectious diseases such as infantile paralysis, measles, diphtheria, whooping cough and tetanus in the newborn has dropped sharply. According to some regional statistics, respiratory diseases, pulmonary tuberculosis, digestive diseases and acute infectious diseases have dropped as the leading causes of death, to be replaced by heart disease, cerebrovascular diseases and cancer. As a result of improvement in the health standard, the mortality rate has dropped from 25 per thousand before liberation to 6.2 per thousand; average life expectancy has risen from 35 to 68, according to statistics compiled from representative regions.

Health work in China has on the whole made rapid progress and achieved great success in the last 30 and more years despite the serious damage it suffered under "Leftist" ideas, particularly at the hands of the Lin Biao and Jiang Qing counter-revolutionary cliques during the "cultural revolution".

From 1949 to 1980, the number of medical and health institutions grew from 3,670 to 180,553 — an increase of 49.2 times, and the number of hospital beds from 80,000 to 1,982,176 — an increase of 24.8 times. The number of hospital beds averaged 0.15 per 1,000 of the population in 1949 and rose to 2.02 in 1980. The following diagrams show the increase in the number of medical institutions, hospitals and beds in the whole country in 1980:

1. Increase in Medical Institutions and Beds

		1949	*1952*	*1965*	*1980*
Total number of medical institutions		3,670	38,987	224,266	180,553
	Hospitals	2,600	3,540	42,711	65,450
	Sanatoria	30	270	887	470
	Clinics	769	29,050	170,430	102,474
	Special disease prevention & treatment centres	11	188	822	1,138

	Health & anti-epidemic stations		147	2,499	3,105
	Maternity & child clinics	9	2,379	2,795	2,610
	Medicine inspection centres	1	12	131	1,213
	Medical research institutes	3	3	94	282
Total number of beds		84,625	230,946	1,033,305	2,184,423
Hospital beds		80,000	160,300	765,558	1,982,176

2. Number of Hospitals and Beds in 1980

	Hospitals	*Beds*
Total	65,450	1,982,176
General hospitals	7,859	941,143
Hospitals of Chinese medicine	678	49,977
Hospitals affiliated to medical colleges or schools	143	62,375

Hospitals for infectious diseases	118	18,580
Mental hospitals	255	49,096
Tuberculosis hospitals	108	25,088
Maternity hospitals	135	11,013
Children's hospitals	24	5,407
Rural commune hospitals	55,413	775,413
Other hospitals	717	44,084

The number of people engaged in medical work increased 6.5 times, from 541,240 in 1949 to 3,534,707 in 1980, while the number of medical technical personnel among them increased 5.5 times, from 505,040 to 2,798,241. The average number of full-time medical technical personnel for 1,000 of the population increased from 0.93 in 1949 to 2.85 in 1980, and the number of doctors from 0.67 to 1.17. The diagram on the next two pages shows the increase in the number of full-time medical personnel in the whole country.

The stress of China's medical and health work is on the rural areas where over 80 per cent of the population live. Tremendous changes have taken place in rural medical service in the last 30 and more years. The 1980 statistics show that China's 2,000-plus counties have

2,377 general hospitals, 2,093 health and anti-epidemic stations and 1,885 maternity and child clinics. Some counties also have hospitals of Chinese medicine, medicine inspection centres, and special disease prevention and treat-

Increase of Full-Time Medical Personnel

		1949	*1952*	*1965*	*1980*
Total number of full-time medical personnel		541,240	818,937	1,872,335	3,534,707
Total number of medical technical personnel		505,040	690,437	1,531,593	2,798,241
	Doctors of Chinese medicine	276,000	306,000	321,430	262,185
	Pharmacists of Chinese medicine		6,536	71,848	106,963
	Doctors of Western medicine	38,000	51,736	188,661	447,288
	Pharmacologists	484	900	8,265	25,241
	Other specialists	391	860	6,476	29,493
	Junior doctors	49,400	66,500	252,713	443,761
	Nurses	32,800	60,900	234,546	465,798

	Midwives	13,900	22,400	45,639	70,843
	Junior pharmacists	2,873	7,071	37,201	83,901
	Other paramedicals	4,304	11,316	49,771	110,132
	Junior medical workers	86,888	156,218	315,045	752,636
Doctors	Doctors of Chinese and Western medicine and junior doctors of Western medicine	363,400	424,236	762,804	1,153,234
	Doctors of Chinese and Western medicine	314,000	357,736	510,091	709,473

ment centres. The country's 50,000-plus people's communes own 55,413 hospitals, and most of the 600,000-plus production brigades in the communes have a co-operative medical service station or a clinic, co-operative medical service having been adopted in 68.8 per cent of them. There are in the rural areas 1.214 million hospital beds, 1.485 million full-time medical technical personnel, 1.463 million barefoot doctors and 2.992 million rural health workers and midwives. The growth of the ranks of the barefoot doctors and the development and consolidation of co-operative medical service have played important roles in overcoming the shortage of doctors and medicine in the countryside.

Most of China's minority nationalities inhabit the remote border regions where there were no doctors, medicine and medical institutions to speak about in the past. The rate of growth in these areas after liberation far exceeds the national average. From 1949 to 1980, the number of medical institutions increased 72.2 times there, with 45.4 times more hospitals, 74.3 times more hospital or sanatorium beds and 91.8 times more full-time medical technical personnel.

Medical Institutions, Beds and Medical Personnel in National Autonomous Areas

	1949	*1952*	*1965*	*1980*
Total number of medical institutions	361	1,176	25,306	26,073
Number of hospitals	230	378	6,275	10,433
Number of hospital and sanatorium beds	3,310	5,711	93,229	245,997
Number of full-time medical technical personnel	3,531	17,877	156,889	324,300

Considerable progress has also been made in medical education and research and other fields of health service, which will be dealt with later.

As an important part of China's socialist construction, medical service is closely related to the health of the people, the strengthening of the country and the regeneration of the nation. The government has decided to strengthen medical and health work in the process of economic readjustment which is unfolding. The guiding principles and main tasks for medical and health work at the present stage are: 1) Continue to place the emphasis on the rural areas and at the same time strengthen work in the factories and mines and in the cities; 2) Continue to implement the policy of prevention first, reinforce public health and anti-epidemic work, launch extensive Patriotic Health Campaigns and make vigorous efforts to prevent and treat those diseases which seriously endanger people's health; 3) Adhere to the policy of simultaneous promotion and long-term support for the three forces — Chinese medicine, Western medicine, and combined Chinese-Western medicine — and develop a medical science that is Chinese; 4) Adopt diverse forms and ways of providing medical service; 5) Strive to give practical guidance for family planning and at the same time do a better work in maternity and child care; 6) Tighten control over pharmacological work to ensure the quality of medicines; 7) Make great efforts to train medical technical and administrative personnel; and 8) Strengthen economic, technological and administrative work in the medical field.

3. PUBLIC HEALTH AND EPIDEMIC PREVENTION

(1) PATRIOTIC HEALTH CAMPAIGN

The Patriotic Health Campaign was begun in 1952 to transform the old China's poor public hygiene. In this campaign, the people of the whole country were encouraged to fight against disease and unhygienic habits, to cultivate gradually a new custom of regarding it as an honour to pay attention to hygiene and a disgrace not to do so, and to improve the general health standard. The campaign was a mass movement aimed at changing the prevailing customs and habits to transform the country; it was also a fundamental measure for implementing the policy of "prevention first" in medical work. The National Committee for Patriotic Health Campaign was once headed by Premier Zhou Enlai, and sub-committees were set up in provinces, municipalities, autonomous regions, prefectures, counties as well as in government departments, enterprises, public institutions, neighbourhood organizations in the cities and agricultural co-operatives in the countryside. Offices were set up or persons appointed to handle the day-to-day work. The principal features of the campaign were: conducting an extensive propaganda and education campaign; mobilizing the people to make a general cleaning of the public places once every season and before the New Year, Spring Festival, International Labour Day and National Day and calling on every household and everybody to improve personal, home and environmental hygiene. At ordinary times, the local committees were responsible for regular work in public hygiene in their localities. The elimination of the "four pests" (rats, flies, mosquitoes and bedbugs) and other germ-carrying insects was also part of the health campaign.

The Patriotic Health Campaign in the rural areas is focused on "two controls" and "five reforms" (control of drinking water and manure; reform of wells, latrines, animal pens, stoves and general environment). With the

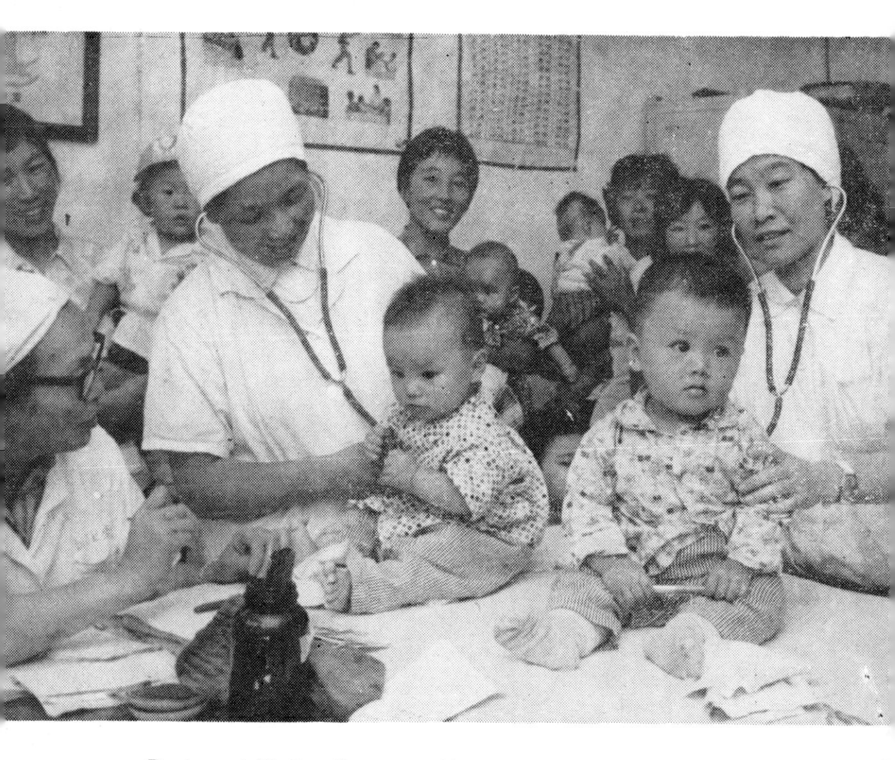

Doctors at Xinjing Commune Hospital in Shanghai County give regular physical check-ups to village children.

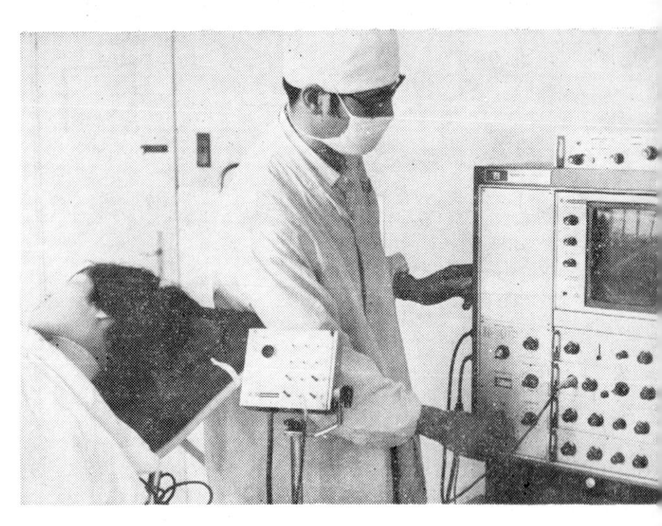

The International Peace Hospital for Maternal and Child Health in Shanghai has an electronic monitoring department to determine the physiological conditions of pre-natal women or women in labour

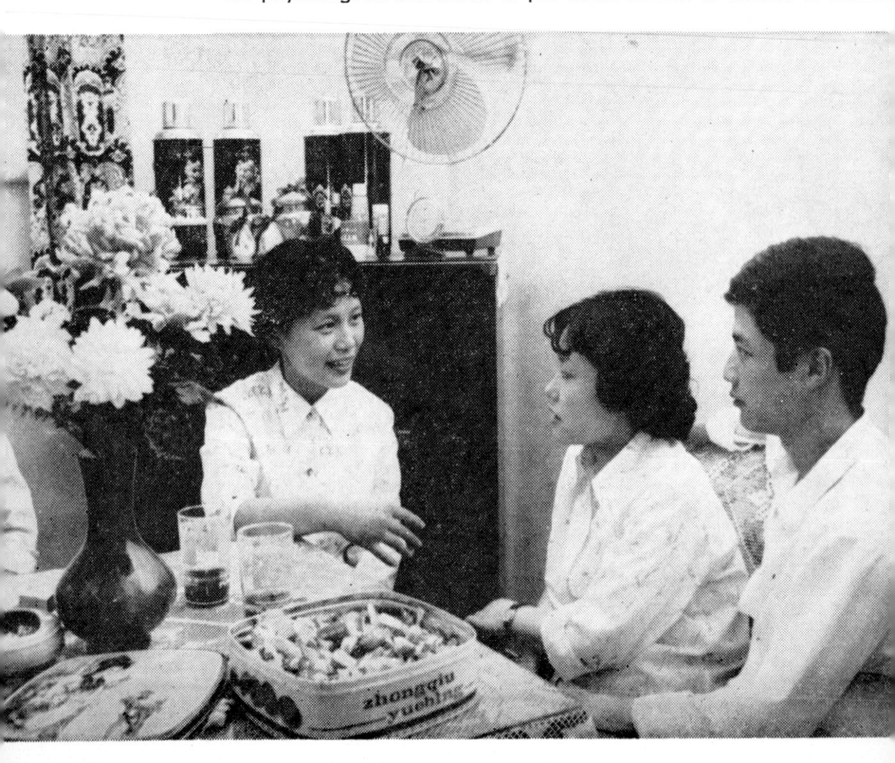

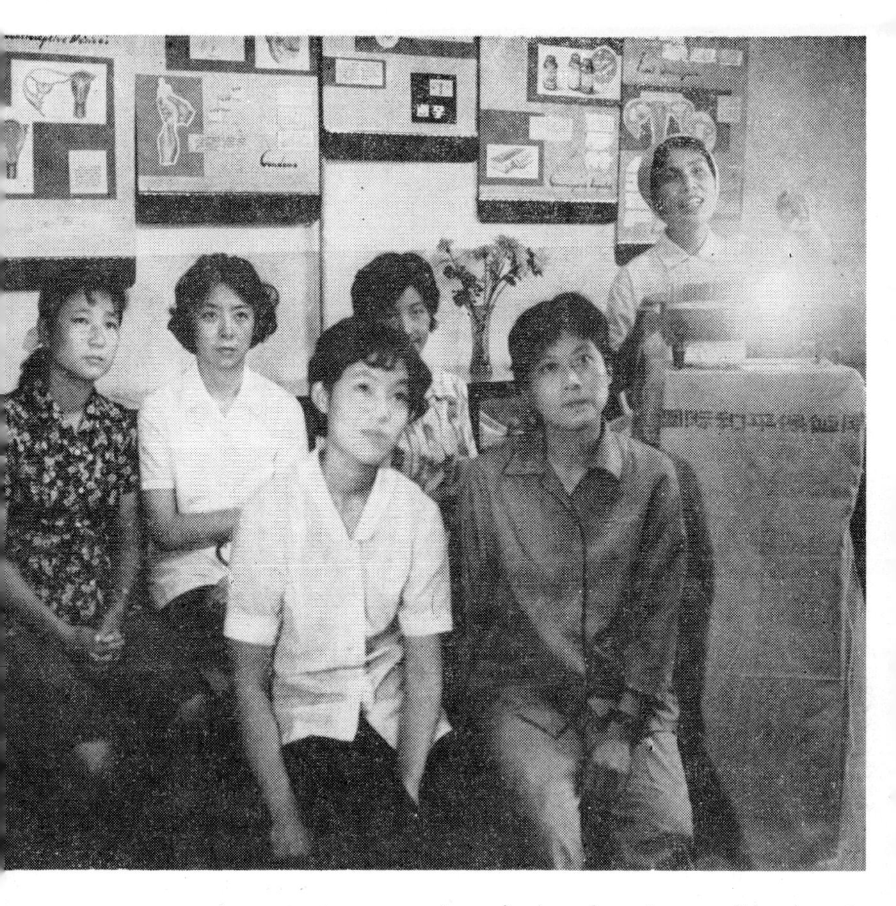

A medical worker gives a slide show to the newlyweds on contraceptive methods.

A doctor visits a newly wedded couple to offer advice on family planning.

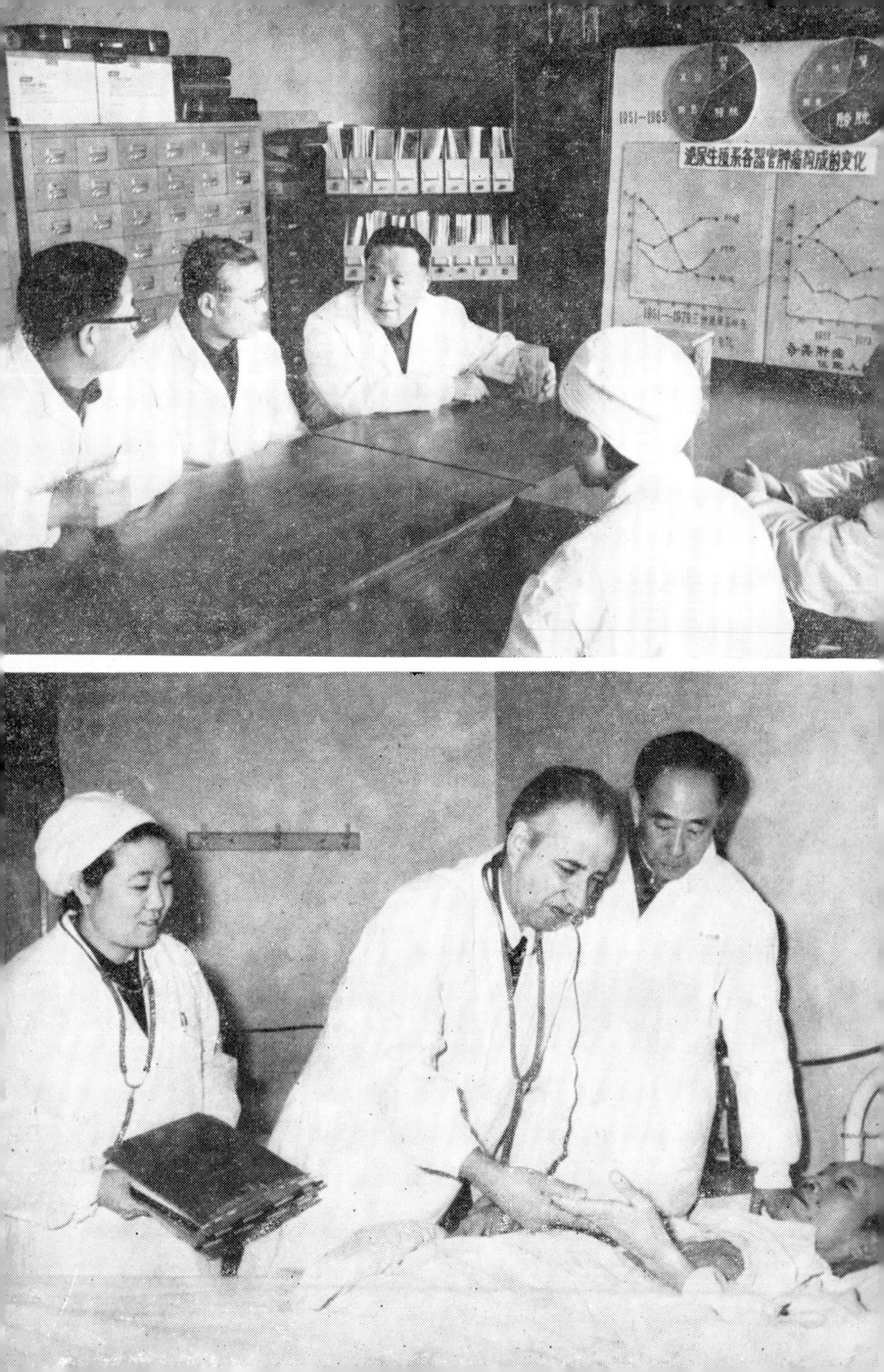
1951—1965
膀胱
泌尿生殖系各器官肿瘤构成的变化

Prof. Wu Jieping (*third from left*), a noted specialist in urological surgery, is seen here discussing the treatment of kidney stones with his colleagues.

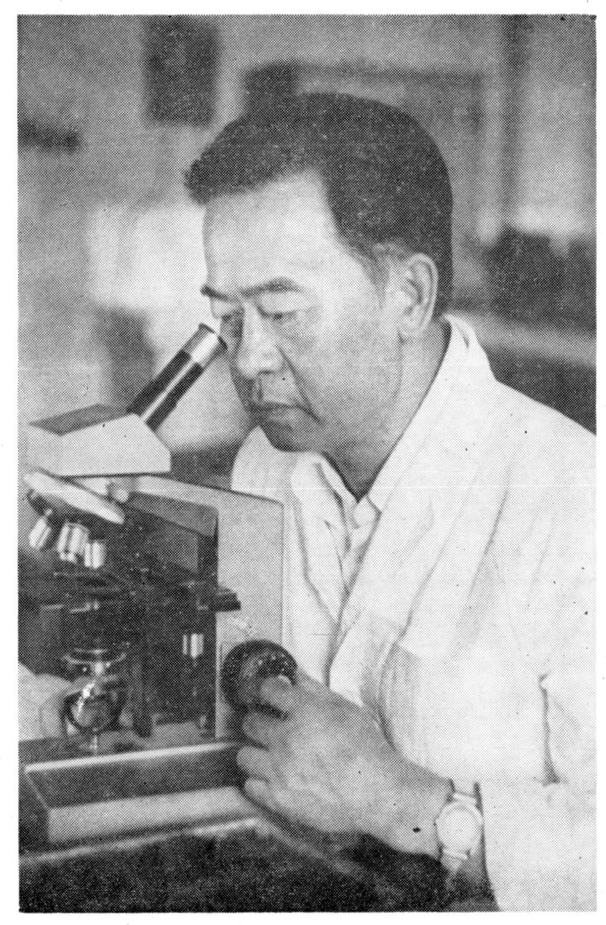

Associate Professor Li Zhenquan of the Zhongshan Medical College of Guangzhou is known for his research of nasopharyngeal carcinoma. His papers have been well received both in China and abroad.

Prof. Hans Müller (*second from left*), Vice-President of the Beijing Medical College, came to China from Germany in the 30s and has been engaged in medical work in China ever since. He is seen here making a round of hospital wards.

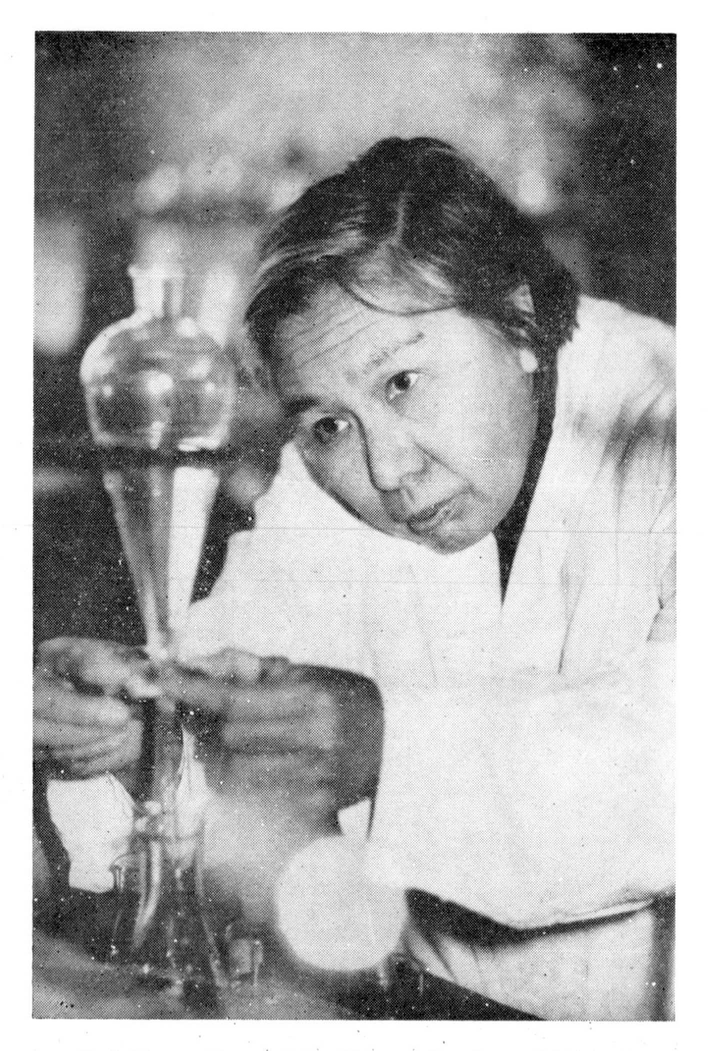

Prof. Huang Liang of the Chinese Academy of Medical Sciences has recently succeeded in finding a new medicine known as harrintonin for treating acute leukemia.

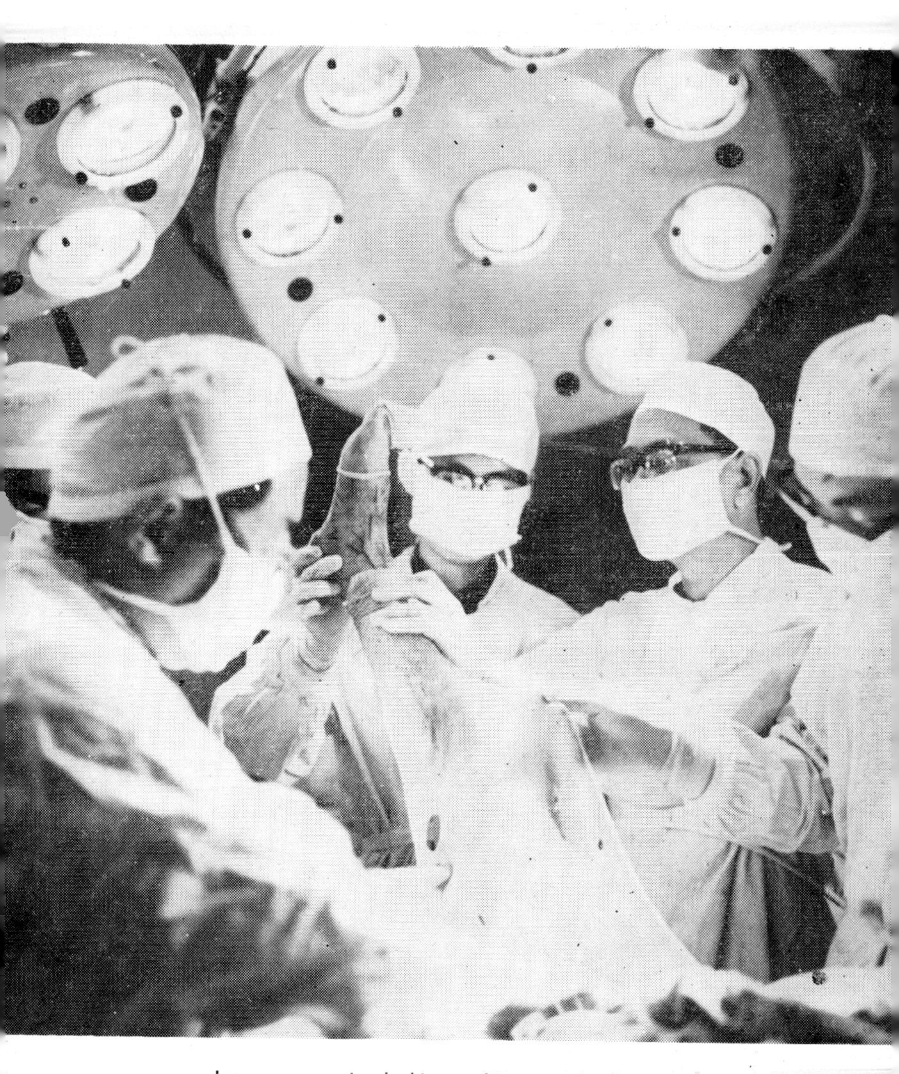

Large-area mixed skin grafting on the leg of a patient suffering from serious burns.

This intracranial stereoscopic locator is a medical instrument newly manufactured in China. It can accurately locate small foreign bodies inside the skull so that operations may be performed in time and without mistake.

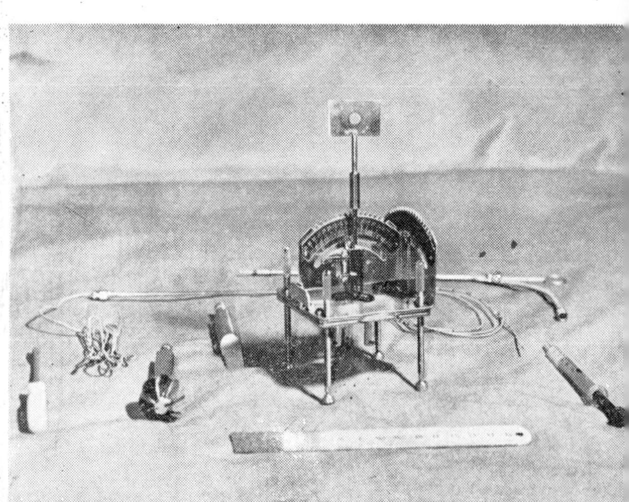

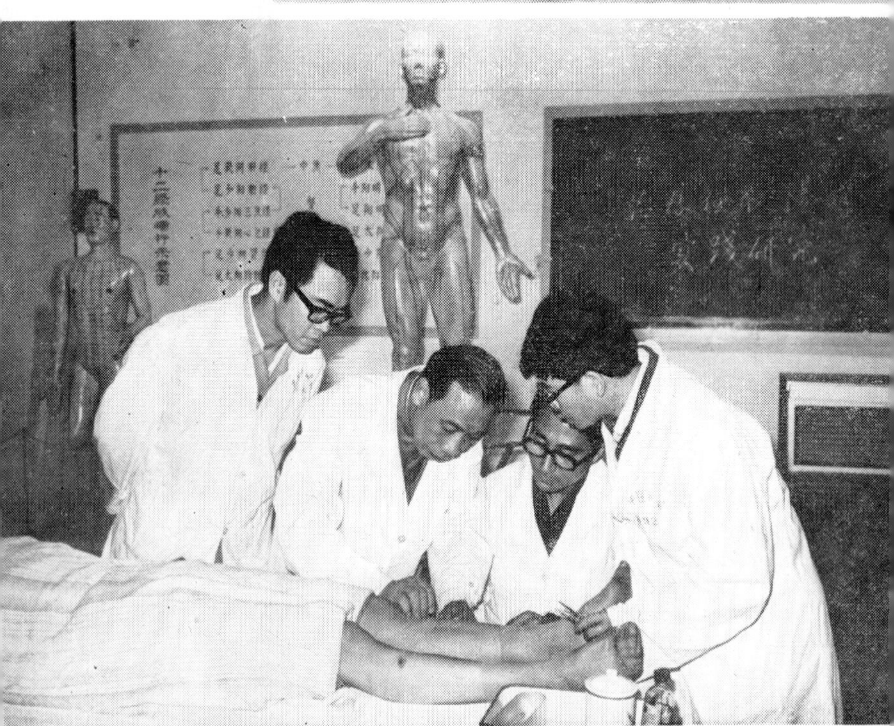

At an acupuncture class in the Guangzhou College of Traditional Chinese Medicine.

construction of irrigation and water conservancy works, the quality of drinking water was improved. Manure was to be collected and dumped into methane-generating pits to help produce methane gas for generating electricity. This also eliminated the breeding grounds of vectors.

The focus of the work in cities and towns was the disposal of garbage, night soil and sewage and the construction of sanitation projects to prevent the contamination of the sources of drinking water and food and the occurrence of diseases.

The Patriotic Health Campaign achieved great successes in the years between 1952 and 1966. Large quantities of pre-liberation garbage and filth were disposed of. Sewage pits were filled up and canals and ditches dredged, decreasing the number of the "four pests" and the incidence of diseases. Paying attention to hygiene gradually became a new social habit. Among the places which became advanced models were Foshan city in Guangdong Province, Qingdao city in Shandong Province, Hangzhou city in Zhejiang Province and Taiyang Village in Jishan County, Shanxi Province. But the campaign came to a standstill in the 10 years of turmoil between 1966 and 1976, resulting in a lowered standard of hygiene and increase of vermin and disease.

The National Committee for Patriotic Health Campaign resumed work in 1978, and in December that year a national conference of the chairmen of the local committees of the Patriotic Health Campaign was convened in Beijing. The conference decided that the campaign was to enter into a new period of development: while continued efforts are to be made to wipe out the "four pests" and diseases and to promote hygiene, a new task — that of fighting against the increasingly serious environmental pollution — must be tackled. The Patriotic Health Campaign was to adopt more scientific methods and become a regular, institutionalized practice. Health work has made remarkable recovery and development in the last few years. In Beijing, for example, the daily disposal of 3,000 tons of garbage and 2,700 tons of night soil has been basically mechanized, and 57 per cent of the production brigades have a tap-water supply. More than four million methane-generating pits have been built in Sichuan Province. The city of Qingdao in Shandong Province has recently completed four huge methane-generating pits having a total capacity of 4,000 cubic metres. A total of 7.29 million latrines have been reconstructed in Shandong, Henan, Heilongjiang and Tianjin. More than 70 per cent of the wells, latrines, animal pens, stoves and general environment in 34 counties in Shanxi Province have been reconstructed.

(2) PREVENTION AND TREATMENT OF INFECTIOUS AND EPIDEMIC DISEASES

After the founding of New China, the People's Government paid particular attention to the prevention and treatment of infectious and epidemic diseases. More than 30 years of efforts participated in by millions of people and medical and health workers have resulted in the elimination or basic elimination of some infectious diseases on a nationwide scale. The incidence and mortality rate of some infectious, parasitic, endemic and occupational diseases have markedly dropped, while those of others have been placed under control. There has been a great improvement in the people's health standard. The People's Government has made particular effort in preventing and treating snail fever (schistosomiasis) and endemic diseases.

Prevention and Treatment of Snail Fever Snail fever has prevailed in China for a long time. A survey made after liberation showed that the disease had spread to 347 counties and cities in south China, namely, in Jiangsu, Zhejiang, Anhui, Jiangxi, Fujian, Shanghai, Hunan, Hubei, Guangxi, Guangdong, Yunnan and Sichuan. By 1979, areas that had been infested by carrier snails at one time or another totalled 13,000 million square metres, and more than 10 million people suffered or had suffered from this disease. Snail fever once caused havoc in the stricken areas of Yujiang County, Jiangxi Province, where 42 villages were virtually wiped out before liberation, with over 25,000 deaths. After the founding of New China, the east China region was the first to set up a prevention and treatment committee and a research committee in the winter of 1949. By the winter of 1955, organizations in all the snail fever areas had been formed for prevention and treatment. Altogether over 16,000 full-time specialists at the end of 1957 and over 13,000 at the end of 1979 were working in this field. Under the leadership of the governments at various levels, these specialists worked with the general population to adopt measures such as killing the carrier snails, treating the disease, and exercising better control over manure and drinking water. By the end of 1979, two-thirds of the infested areas had been cleared of carrier snails and two-thirds of the patients fully cured. Snail fever had been basically eliminated in over 200 counties and cities, and in Guangdong, Jiangsu, Guangxi, Fujian and Shanghai.

Prevention and Treatment of Endemic Diseases These diseases like endemic goitre, Keshan disease, Kaschin-Beck disease and endemic fluorosis are found in varying degrees in 16 provinces, municipalities and autonomous regions of northern China. The National Programme of Agricultural Development promulgated in 1958 listed endemic goitre, Keshan disease and Kaschin-Beck disease as afflictions to be actively prevented and treated. A national leading group for preventing and treating endemic diseases was formed in March 1960 as were organizations and teams of specialists in all the northern provinces, prefectures, counties and cities where such diseases occur. An endemic disease science committee was set up in June 1979 to reinforce related research.

Endemic goitre. Goitre, an enlargement of the thyroid gland, is caused by lack of iodine in the natural surroundings (water and earth) and food (vegetables, grain, etc.). The offspring of goitre patients may be congenital cretins characterized by dementia, dwarfism and paralysis. Endemic goitre can be prevented and cured by using iodized salt, orally administering potassium iodide, injecting iodized oil or by traditional Chinese medicine. Large numbers of patients have been cured, and some counties and cities have placed this disease under control and succeeded in preventing new cases from breaking out.

Keshan disease. First found in Keshan County, Heilongjiang Province, in 1907, Keshan disease is an endemic myocardiac ailment which causes heart failure, breathing difficulties, dropsy and abdominal distension. Another outbreak of the disease, which entails a high rate of mortality, took place in 1935, and as no definite causes had been found, it was named Keshan disease. In the early post-liberation days, the mortality rate in acute and serious cases was as high as over 85 per cent, and the disease spread to 205 counties and districts in 11 provinces.

Since 1960, encouraging results have been achieved in treating patients with intravenous injections of large doses of Vitamin C. Oral administration of sodium selenite which began in 1965 has also brought satisfactory result. Early diagnosis and early treatment have gradually brought down the incidence and mortality rate of Keshan disease. Acute or subacute cases of the disease have not occurred for five and even 10 years running in one-fifth of the stricken areas.

Kaschin-Beck disease. The cause of this disease characterized by a swelling of the joints is still not clear. Since liberation, hypotheses and methods of prevention and treatment have been suggested by the public health, water conservancy and geological departments following joint studies and investigations. The number of patients has dropped in most of the stricken areas as a result of some preventive and curative measures.

Endemic fluorosis. Chronic fluorosis is caused by a high fluoride content in drinking water, food grain and vegetables. The damage is chiefly done to the bones, resulting in dental fluorosis or, in more serious cases, fluorosis of the bones. Intensive study of this disease began in the 1950s, and in 1977 it was listed as an important disease to be prevented and treated. Effective results have been achieved by sinking wells, drawing spring water for drinking and eliminating fluoride in the water by chemical or physical methods. Some of the affected areas are now free from fluoride poisoning. Efforts are being made in various localities to find from among Chinese and Western medicines the most effective cure for fluorosis patients.

(3) POPULARIZATION OF HEALTH AND MEDICAL KNOWLEDGE

The national and local newspapers, magazines, radio and TV stations and publishing houses regularly engage in promoting health and medical knowledge. News and feature articles about health and medical work regularly appear in the newspapers. The Central People's Broadcasting Station runs a "Pay Attention to Hygiene" programme, and the China Central Television has a "Health and Hygiene" programme. *Health Journal* published by the Ministry of Public Health has a circulation of 340,000. The People's Health Publishing House puts out an average of 140 books a year, in addition to the 102 journals published by organizations under the Ministry of Public Health. Many more journals and popular magazines and booklets disseminating medical knowledge are being published by the provinces, municipalities and autonomous regions.

China observed International Children's Year and World Health Day by launching publicity campaigns against smoking and for the protection of children's health. With the approval of the State Council, the Ministries of Public Health, Finance, Agriculture and Light Industry jointly issued the "Circular on Publicizing the Harm of Smoking and on Controlling Smoking" in July 1979 and banned smoking in hospitals, conference halls, theatres, cinemas, kindergartens and buses. College and school students are prohibited from smoking by school authorities.

4. MATERNITY AND CHILD CARE

Special importance is given to maternity and child care in China's medical service. A network for protecting the health of mother and child has been established in all the cities and countryside. The Ministry of Public Health has a bureau devoted to maternity and child care. A paediatric research institute operates under the Chinese Academy of Medical Sciences. In the various provinces, municipalities and autonomous regions, besides gynaecological, obstetric and paediatric departments in general hospitals, there are maternity hospitals, children's hospitals and maternity and child health centres. Maternity and child health centres, stations or groups also exist in city districts, counties, rural people's communes and production brigades. In those production brigades where there is no health station, the work is looked after by barefoot doctors, medical attendants or midwives. Figures of 1980 showed that there were 24 children's hospitals, 135 maternity and child health centres and 2,610 maternity and child health stations in the whole country. The figures also showed that there were over 50,000 doctors of gynaecology, obstetrics and paediatrics, and 70,000 full-time and 600,000 part-time midwives.

This is a far cry from the situation over 30 years ago.

Popularizing Modern Methods of Delivery In old China, the mortality rate was high for both infants and women during childbirth. Immediately after the founding of the People's Republic, the introduction of modern methods of delivery and training of midwives and other medical workers for women and children brought about a remarkable fall in the mortality rate. The infant mortality rate in Beijing city proper, for example, dropped from 117.6 per thousand in 1949 to about 10 per thousand in 1980, while the mortality rate of women both before and after delivery fell from 7 per thousand to 0.13 per thousand in the corresponding period.

Health Service for Women Health service for women aims mainly at preventing diseases during menstruation, pregnancy, childbirth, nursing and menopause. The work has been extensively promoted. Health service during pregnancy and childbirth emphasizes early check-ups to prevent complications such as gestosis and high blood pressure, and to prevent difficult childbirth by the early discovery of abnormal foetal position. Some cities have adopted a systematic method of care for expectant mothers, which includes detailed registration and home visits at regular intervals. According to government stipulations, working women are given special protection. Women peasants, for example, are excused from working in the paddy-fields during menstruation and given light work during pregnancy. Working mothers with nursing babies are given time during the working hours to feed their babies. The above measures have greatly reduced the incidence of disease and the mortality rate of women during pregnancy and childbirth.

General Check-Ups and Treatment of Women's Common Diseases A general check-up and treatment of cervical carcinoma which began in 1958 in the big cities has been extended to districts and counties with better medical facilities, markedly reducing its incidence and increasing the rate of cure. General gynaecological examinations are being conducted in many areas using such methods as ultraviolet fluorescent examination and cytological examination of the cervix. Metroptosis (prolapse of the womb) and urinary fistula are common among women living in remote mountain areas. Prevention and treatment teams were formed in 1978 for training technical personnel and giving free medical treatment for these complaints.

Health Service for Children Smallpox was wiped out in China in 1960, and diphtheria and poliomyelitis were placed under control. The universal BCG and diphtheria vaccinations among children in the cities and countryside and preventive and curative measures against measles have combined to greatly lower the incidence rate of these diseases. For better child care, a card system has been introduced in some cities and rural areas where regular physical check-ups are given to the children and, where necessary, home visits are made and treatment provided. In addition, health service in kindergartens and nurseries has been continually improved.

Family Planning To give practical guidance in family planning has always been an important regular responsibility of the medical departments. Different contraceptive measures according to each person's particular situation are encouraged by medical institutions at all levels, which also work to promote scientific understanding about family planning, supervise and plan the training of technical personnel, engage in scientific research and popularize new methods and techniques. As part of the concern about bearing sound offspring, knowledge about hereditary factors affecting birth has been emphasized in recent years. The related departments have begun to investigate hereditary diseases, and some medical and health service units have set up heredity consulting departments which can help ascertain the physical conditions of the foetus. As family planning has developed, proper attention has been given to the new situation and solving new problems, such as improving the health care and education of the only child.

5. ENVIRONMENT AND HEALTH

Environmental Protection As China's modernization started rather late, environmental protection did not draw much attention until the early 1970s. The First National Conference on Environmental Protection held in 1973 adopted the Draft Regulations Concerning Environmental Protection and Improvement. The following year saw the formation of an umbrella organization comprising responsible members of the State Council's departments of industry, communications, agriculture, forestry, public health, oceanology and education, to plan and supervise environmental protection on a nationwide scale. Environmental control organizations were then set up in all the provinces, municipalities, autonomous regions, larger cities and important counties and enterprises, and for major bodies of water. As the "cultural revolution" was then under way, progress was slow and results far from satisfactory. Today, all the 216 large and medium-sized cities in the country suffer from different degrees of pollution and 15 of the 27 principal rivers are rather badly polluted. In September 1979, the Standing Committee of the National People's Congress promulgated the Environmental Protection Law (for Trial Implementation), and a series of specific rules and regulations suited to local conditions were adopted in 1980 by the people's congress standing committees and people's governments of the provinces, municipalities and autonomous regions and many cities to help implement the above-mentioned law. Among the research institutions of environmental science that had come into existence by the end of 1980 were: the Research Academy of Environmental Science, the Institute of Environmental Chemistry under the Chinese Academy of Sciences, 27 provincial-level research institutes of environmental protection, seven special environmental protection research institutes of the chemical, metallurgical and other industries, and the China Society of Environmental Science. Over a dozen journals of environmental protection are published in various places. As many as 6,000 scientists are making fairly rapid headway in their study of environmental social sciences, environmental quality, the technique of pollution control, environmental chemistry, biology, medicine, acoustics, and noise control. There are now 354 monitoring stations across the length and breadth of the country, staffed by over 6,800 technicians, in addition to those set up by the departments of industry, communications, agriculture, forestry, foreign trade, aquatic production, etc., and by many major industrial enterprises. Education in environmental protection is given at school and in the community and includes in-service training of working personnel. China has attended a number of UNO-sponsored environmental protection conferences, run a methane-generating class for the UNEP (United Nations Environment Programme) and carried out international exchanges and co-operation in environmental protection. Much has been done to create a better environment for people to live in and for industry, agriculture, forestry, fishery and animal husbandry. Today, the environmental quality in some places already measures up to the state-stipulated standards and in other places it is basically under control. But much more effort has to be made to improve environmental quality as a whole.

Health Inspection The health departments are also doing a tremendous amount of work in exercising control over health standards in working conditions and in general environment, in hygiene in food and the schools, and in radioactivity levels. The Ministry of Public Health has laid down standards for industrial production, diagnosis standards of work-related diseases, hygienic standards for 110 types of food, and stipulated protective measures against and control over radioactive materials. To guard against food contamination, the Ministry has laid down 75 permanent and provisional state standards for 18 categories of food, including grain, oil, meat, eggs and some aquatic products, and 36 state standards for food additives. These standards are based on investigation and study and scientific experiments and nearly 100 million figures obtained from inspection and monitoring in the whole country. The State Council promulgated in 1979 the Regulations of Food Hygiene of the People's Republic of China.

Study of Pollution and People's Health This study, which began in 1978, is sponsored by the Ministry of Public Health and undertaken by the Health Research Institute of the Chinese Academy of Medical Sciences and the bureaux of public health of the provinces and municipalities concerned. It involves an investigation into epidemics, a quick screening of cancer-causing pollutants, study of the relationship between atmospheric pollution and the occurrence of lung cancer (participated in by 24 cities and the prefecture of Xuanwei in Yunnan Province), the effect of the pollution of the Bohai and Huanghai seas by heavy metals on people's health (participated in by the provinces and cities on the shores of the two seas), the mercurial pollution of the Songhua River on the health of the fishermen, the effect of a minimal amount of organic chloride in drinking water on health, etc. Progress has been made in all these studies. Some scientists have put forward a theory on the carcinogenicity of polycyclic aromatic hydrocarbons, and further studies are being made on the subject.

Environmental Hygiene in the Countryside As many kinds of insecticides tend to endanger people's health by contaminating soil, water sources and crops, China is steadily adopting biological means to combat insect pests. Satisfactory results have been achieved, for example, in the use of trichogramma, ladybug and *Goldaugen* against pests of grain, cotton and oil-bearing crops and forest trees. Good results have also been achieved in the use of micro-organisms including *Sporeine* against maize borer, pine moth and rice plant skipper, and in the use of antibiotics such as jinggangmycin and kasukamycin against sheath and culm blight of rice, rice blast and apple rot. An investigation conducted in 1979 in 26 provinces, municipalities and autonomous regions showed that a great number of the natural enemies of insect pests can be found in China. In Hunan Province alone, for instance, there are 113 paddyfield spiders that can be used to kill some insect pests.

As plant stalks, leaves and wood are still the chief sources of fuel in Chinese countryside, fewer and fewer stalks are ploughed in after harvest to maintain the fertility of the soil. The indiscriminate clearing of forests has worsened soil erosion, adversely affected the climate and gravely disrupted the natural environment. Great efforts are being made to popularize small hydro-power stations and methane-generating pits as ways of solving this energy problem in the countryside. Small hydro-power stations have been built in more than 1,500 of the 2,000-plus counties in the whole country. Methane generation has been popularized in more than 20 counties and is being spread to many more. Manure, garbage, weeds and other organic matter are placed in the methane-generating pits to ferment. The easily decomposed part becomes methane, which can be used as fuel or for generating electricity, and the not so easily decomposed part becomes good-quality compost. In the process of fermentation, most of the eggs of liver flukes, hookworms and roundworms and many germs are killed, greatly reducing the incidence of some infectious diseases in rural areas.

Control of Industrial Pollution Industries are the chief culprits behind pollution of air and water in the cities and countryside. To put new sources of pollution under control, the government requires that all enterprises under construction, expansion or reconstruction incorporate environmental protection devices into their projects. In October 1978, the government set a deadline for 167 factories and mines to adjust their 261 sources of pollution before 1982. By the end of 1980, some 143, or 54.8 per cent, of these sources had been placed under control through a variety of methods including comprehensive utilization, turning harm into benefit, technical reform and stricter control. For example, the waste gas discharged by oil refineries is recovered to make synthetic fibres, synthetic rubber, plastics and chemical fertilizer.

The residue from some factories and mines is used for making chemical fertilizer, cement, bricks and refractory materials. The chemical, pharmaceutical and light industrial departments are extracting and recovering hundreds of products from waste water. The industrial departments are popularizing the use of non-mercurial meters, non-cyanic methods of plating, fermentive methods of removing hair from animal skins and techniques for treating and recycling waste water in the oilfields. Coal-burning boilers have been rebuilt to control smoke and coal dust pollution, and some factories have been moved to sparsely populated areas. Rivers, lakes and seas that have already been polluted by industries or oilfields are continually monitored, and measures are being taken to restore them to their natural condition. These measures have ensured the quality of drinking water, food and air, and reduced the incidence of diseases.

Urban Environmental Protection Multiple efforts are being made to protect the environment in the cities, particularly cities which have been designated to receive special protection, including Beijing, Tianjin, Shanghai, Hangzhou, Suzhou, Lanzhou, Shenyang and Guilin. Protective measures, for example, are responsible for the quality of the water in Beijing's three large reservoirs — the Guanting, Miyun and Huairou — never having dropped below the standard set by the government for sources of drinking water. The Changhe, Tonghui and five other rivers were once badly contaminated by 401 serious sources of pollution. Now 324 of these sources have been neutralized, greatly lessening the pollution. Some 86 per cent of the 5,095 boilers in the city area have been rebuilt and no longer bellow smoke and coal dust. Except for winter when central heating is on, the quality of the atmosphere in Beijing proper basically meets the standard set by the government. A number of noisy factories have been moved out of the populated areas. In the city of Hangzhou, environmental protection is focused on and around the West Lake, one of China's best-known resort areas. The measures taken include reinforcing 20-plus kilometres of lake shore, laying 9.4 kilometres of sewage pipes and building eight lakeside pump-houses to prevent sewage from flowing into the lake. The 56 pleasure boats plying the lake are now operated by battery instead of diesel engines. To control noise, trucks are prohibited from entering the scenic areas, and diesel trucks are banned from the city area. Smoke and dust elimination devices have been installed on all the 55 boilers in use by the various establishments around the lake. Tea houses now use natural gas instead of coal. A factory that was harmful to West Lake scenery has been moved away. The result is a more peaceful and hygienic environment for both residents and tourists.

6. CHINESE MEDICINE AND PHARMACOLOGY

(1) DEVELOPMENT OF CHINESE MEDICINE

As stated in Section 1, Chinese medicine has a rich store of practical experience and theoretical knowledge. Immediately after the founding of New China, Chairman Mao Zedong emphasized that "it is necessary to unite with doctors of traditional Chinese medicine, improve their skills, encourage them to work well and bring traditional Chinese medicine into play; only then can we shoulder the tremendous task of looking after the health of several hundred millions of people". Later, Chinese medical workers were called on to investigate the whys and hows of traditional Chinese medicine from a modern scientific point of view and develop a new Chinese medicine which combines Western medicine. Great progress was made between 1949 and 1965 in promoting traditional Chinese medicine and combining it with Western medicine. By the end of 1965, there were already over 280,000 doctors of Chinese medicine in the whole country working in medical institutions owned either by the whole people or by collectives, and their social status had been raised considerably. The Academy of Traditional Chinese Medicine and 21 colleges of Chinese medicine were set up and a number of hospitals of traditional medicine established or reinforced. More than 5,600 were graduated from colleges of Chinese medicine and over 59,000 apprentices trained. Many doctors of traditional medicine received further training during this period. More than 4,400 doctors of Western medicine were released from their regular jobs to study Chinese medicine. Among those who studied for two years were over 2,000 who were senior members of their profession. Some important results were achieved in the study of combining Chinese and Western medicine. Ancient Chinese medical books and the experience of well-known doctors of Chinese medicine were studied and put in order. At the same time, a large number of books and textbooks of Chinese medicine and pharmacology were published.

Chinese medicine and pharmacology also suffered disruption during the "cultural revolution" and did not begin to recover and develop anew until a few years ago. The First National Symposium on Traditional Chinese Medicine was held in Beijing in May 1979. A grand gathering in the history of the development of Chinese medicine, it was participated in by over 380 delegates who were experts of Chinese medicine or combined Chinese and Western medicine, and by doctors of Tibetan, Mongolian or Uygur medicine. The symposium received over 1,300 papers which reflected new developments in clinical and research work. A resolution for the setting up of the All-China Society of Traditional Chinese Medicine was adopted at the conference. A national symposium on acupuncture anaesthesia was convened in June 1979 to discuss what had been accomplished in scientific research in this particular field. It was favourably received by both the Chinese and foreign specialists who attended. Figures of 1980 showed that there were 678 hospitals and 22 colleges of Chinese medicine, 20 secondary schools and 47 research institutes of Chinese medicine and pharmacology, 262,185 doctors of Chinese medicine and 106,963 traditional pharmacists. Societies of traditional Chinese medicine at various levels had been founded or had resumed activity, and journals of Chinese medicine were being published or had resumed publication. Many provinces, municipalities and autonomous regions ran classes for the training of teachers and for advanced studies in Chinese medicine to raise the professional skill of the doctors and pharmacists. A national working conference on Chinese and Chinese-Western medicine was held in March 1980. The conference advocated the long-term co-existence and simultaneous development of the three branches of medicine — Chinese, Western and Chinese-Western — to promote the modernization of medical sciences and develop a new medicine and pharmacology with Chinese characteristics. The main points of the policy towards traditional Chinese medicine are: to work hard to carry forward, further discover, sort out and improve Chinese medicine and pharmacology; to unite with and rely on doctors of Chinese medicine to develop and raise the standard of Chinese medicine; to organize doctors of Western medicine to learn and study Chinese medicine and combine it and Western medicine; and to adopt advanced technology to modernize traditional Chinese medicine.

(2) NEW ACHIEVEMENTS IN CHINESE AND CHINESE-WESTERN MEDICINE

Chinese medicine has its own system of theories, therapeutic principles and methods of treatment. Efforts to study and explain them from a modern approach and in connection with clinical experience have led to some new successes. In acupuncture and moxibustion, for example, a number of new acupuncture points and new methods of treatment have been discovered so that more than 300 types of ailments can be treated now, 100 of which with good or very good results, including coronary heart disease, acute bacterial dysentry, gall stones, neural paralysis, diseases of the ear, eye, lip, nose and tongue. This method can also be used in inducing labour and correcting the position of a foetus. The pain-killing effect induced by acupuncture in many clinical instances led to the use of acupuncture anaesthesia in surgical operations. The patient under acupuncture anaesthesia remains conscious, is able to co-operate with the doctor during the operation, suffers less post-operative pains and recovers faster. Acupuncture anaesthesia is now being more and more widely applied and its theory more thoroughly studied. It is now extensively used in operations on the head, neck, chest and abdomen and has achieved successful results in more difficult operations such as cardiac surgery under direct vision with extracorporeal circulation and replantation of severed limbs.

Qigong (breathing exercises) therapy has achieved remarkable results in promoting health and in the treatment of diseases. Doing *qigong* exercises not only keeps one in good health, energetic in spirit, but has also restored to health some patients suffering from severe diseases. People both in China and abroad are increasingly interested in the study of these exercises. Such study, focused on the question of what is *qi*, has yielded preliminary results. Chinese methods of bonesetting have also been studied by modern medical knowledge and method which has brought about new interpretations in theory. Fairly satisfactory results have been obtained in the treatment, mainly by massage, of atlanto-axial subluxation, ailments of the cervical vertebrae, disorder of the posterior lumbar vertebral joint, prolapse of the lumbar intervertebral disc, injury of nervi glutaeus superior, omalgia and some other soft tissue injuries. The treatment of fractures by combined Chinese and Western therapeutic method has a higher rate of cure than by Chinese or Western method alone. Successes have been achieved in the use of splints, early exercise of fractured limbs and internal and external administration of Chinese medicine to hasten the healing of the injured bones by relieving pain and local swellings, helping circulation and accelerating bone growth.

(3) CHINESE PHARMACOLOGY

The Chinese Pharmaceutical Corporation was set up in 1955. In 1958, the State Council issued the Directive for Developing the Production of Chinese Medicinal Materials. The Ministry of Public Health and the Ministry of Commerce jointly convened in 1977 a conference for exchanging experience in the growing and gathering of Chinese medicinal herbs and the manufacture and use of medicines produced with them as raw materials. The State Council approved in 1978 the Summary of the National Conference on the Production of Chinese Medicinal Materials. The production, research and marketing departments in various areas have done a great deal in promoting the development of Chinese pharmacology.

Chinese Medicinal Materials According to 1979 statistics, medicinal plants were grown on 6.07 million mu* of land in the old and new production centres, nearly three times the area in 1957. In the same year, a total of 980 million yuan worth of medicinal materials, over three times that of 1957, was purchased by state-owned pharmaceutical companies. Compared with 1949, the output of such famous medicinal plants as angelica of Gansu, coptis of Sichuan and Hubei, and ginseng of the northeast doubled or was several times higher in 1980. Elevated gastrodia, pinellia, balloonflower and 53 other medicinal herbs which formerly grew only in the wild are now being cultivated. The cultivating areas for over 100 kinds of medicinal plants, including *dangshen* (*Condonopsis pilosula*), *fuling* (*Poris cocos*), chrysanthemum and Chinese yam, have been enlarged. China used to have to import such medicinal materials as Radix Aucklandiae, Fructus Chebulae, bezoar, borneol, Concretio Silicea Bambusae, amber and pearl. Enough of these are now being produced not only to meet domestic needs, but also to be

* One mu equals 1/15 hectare.

exported. There are now altogether more than 5,000 types of Chinese medicinal herbs in use and most of them are available at a trifling price. The development of Chinese medicinal materials has a special significance for improving the medical and health conditions of China's large rural population and for consolidating and expanding rural co-operative medical service.

Fruitful results have also been obtained in the studies of the effects of Chinese medicinal materials. For example, a large number of Chinese herbal medicines have been screened for their anti-cancer properties. More than 100 types of herbs are now being tested in the laboratory or through clinical means. The "Jiangyaling" hypertension pills, or verticil, made from *Rauwoflia verticillata* is now in common clinical use. Repeated tests show that the root of red-rooted salvia, the root of kudzu vine, the rhizome of *chuanxiong* and pseudo-ginseng increase coronary circulation and reduce oxygen consumption by the heart, and consequently they are effective to a certain extent in the treatment of coronary disease and angina pectoris. Both the extract of artemisia and an extract from B-dichroine are new effective medicines for malaria.

Patent Chinese Medicines Chinese medicines traditionally have been prepared in the forms of pills, powder, oilment, pellets, tincture, drinks, syrup, lumps and gelatin. Now they are also prepared as injections, tablets, dissolubles and sprays. In 1980, about 3,000 patent Chinese medicines in more than 20 forms of preparation were on the market.

Among the many nationally famous Chinese pharmaceutical works are Tong Ren Tang in Beijing, Da Ren Tang in Tianjin, Hu Qingyu Tang in Hangzhou and Lei Yunshang Tang in Suzhou. There are over 100 patent preparations of famous brands, some of which have very long histories. The Angong Bezoar Pellet, Black Chicken and White Phoenix Pellet and Tiger Bone Wine of Beijing's Tong Ren Tang, Liushen Pills of Shanghai and of Suzhou's Lei Yunshang Tang, Baiyao Powder of Yunnan, and Guilingji and Dingkundan of Taigu in Shanxi are also well known abroad. An increasing number of new patent Chinese medicines are being made. Among the over 500 new medicines that appeared between 1961 and 1980 are some which have proved remarkably effective — an anaesthetic injection for abdominal operations, Bezoar Anti-Hypertension Pills, and Yufeng Ningxin Pills (also for lowering high blood pressure), Zhongjiefeng Tablets which reduce inflammation, and Subingdi Pills and Guanxin Suhe Pills for heart disease.

The output and sales of patent Chinese medicines have increased phenomenally. Compared with 1955, the output in 1978 increased 92 times, domestic sales value 131 times and export 22 times.

(4) MEDICINE AND PHARMACOLOGY OF MINORITY NATIONALITIES

Tibetan Medicine Tibetan medicine and pharmacology occupy an important place among those of China's minority nationalities. A hospital of Tibetan medicine was set up in Lhasa, seat of the Tibet Autonomous Region, after liberation to provide medical services for the masses of the Tibetan people. The Tibet Medical College was founded in 1978 with departments of Tibetan medicine and pharmacology. A number of Tibetan medical books, including the *Selected Writings on Tibetan Medicine and*

Pharmacology by Luosang Quepei and *Clinical Notes of Tibetan Medicine* by Yundan Jiacuo, have been edited and published. *The Commonly Used Tibetan Herbal Medicines* and *An Illustrated Dictionary of Medicinal Materials Found on the Qinghai-Tibet Plateau* have been published in Tibetan and Han editions with the aim of clarifying the confusion in the names and uses of Tibetan medicines. A *Tibetan Pharmacopoeia* was jointly compiled and published by the six provinces and autonomous regions where Tibetan medicine is practised. The clinical experience of veteran doctors of Tibetan medicine is being summarized and analysed. Five veteran doctors of Tibetan Medicine in Xiahe County, Gansu Province, co-authored a book entitled *Si Xu Bao Ji,* in which they summed up their long years of clinical experience. Progress has also been made in the research and production of Tibetan medicines some of which are effective in curing gastric ulcer, hypertension, tracheitis and arthritis.

Mongolian Medicine Mongolian and Tibetan schools of medicine are based on similar theory. In 1958 a department of Chinese (Mongolian) medicine was set up at the Inner Mongolia Medical College. The Inner Mongolia College of Mongolian Medicine and the Inner Mongolia Research Institute of Chinese (Mongolian) Medicine were established in 1979. Recently published books of Mongolian medicine include the *Illustrated Catalogue of Herbal Medicines* and *A Treasure Book of Medicine.* The Tibetan *Four-Volume Medical Encyclopaedia* has been translated and published in Mongolian.

Uygur Medicine This school of medicine was created by the Uygur people who drew on the Han Chinese, Tibetan and Arab schools of medicine. There are three hospitals of Uygur medicine in the Xinjiang Uygur

Autonomous Region. A number of books of Uygur medicine are available.

Tai Medicine An enormous body of medical literature, especially simple prescriptions and methods of healing which are scattered among the Tai people in Yunnan Province, has been preserved. The Xishuangbanna Autonomous Prefecture has organized a research team to seek out and catalogue the Tai medical traditions. It has so far discovered that more than 1,400 medicines are being used among the Tai people.

Yi Medicine A medical book written in the Yi language over 400 years ago (during the reign of Jiajing in the Ming Dynasty) which was discovered in 1979 in Chuxiong County, Yunnan Province, proves that Yi medicine has had a long history. This book of 5,000 Yi characters records commonly used medicines and simple methods of treating 54 kinds of disease. Efforts have been made in recent years to collect and sort out Yi medical records and experience.

7. MEDICAL EDUCATION AND RESEARCH

(1) MEDICAL EDUCATION

Medical education, important in continuously raising standards of medical service and medical personnel, is conducted in China along three lines: secondary, higher and post-graduate. In the countryside, there are also training schools and classes for medical attendants.

Higher Medical Education Available 1980 figures show that medical education was offered at 112 institutes of higher learning in the whole country, including 109 medical and pharmaceutical colleges and 3 universities each having a medical college or department. There are 63 colleges of Western medicine, 22 colleges of traditional Chinese medicine, 2 pharmaceutical colleges and 25 junior medical colleges, staffed by 30,808 full-time teachers in all. Between 1949 and 1980, some 406,000 graduated from medical or pharmaceutical colleges, 43.7 times more than the number of graduates between 1928 and 1947. The medical and pharmaceutical colleges in China offer five college courses lasting eight, six, five, four or three years, and three graduate courses lasting four, three or two years. Among the 112 institutes, 99 are under the guidance of the provincial, municipal and autonomous regional governments or central departments. The 13 institutes under the leadership mainly of the Ministry of Public Health are: China Capital Medical University, Beijing Medical College, Beijing College of Traditional Chinese Medicine, Shanghai First Medical College, Zhongshan Medical College, the medical colleges of Sichuan, Wuhan, Hunan and Shandong, China Medical University, Bethune Medical University, Xi'an Medical College and Guangzhou College of Traditional Chinese Medicine.

Secondary Medical Education According to the 1980 figures, there were 553 secondary medical schools in the whole country staffed by some 22,835 full-time teachers. These include 443 health schools, 78 nursing schools, 1 midwife-training school, 22 schools of traditional Chinese medicine and pharmacology, 6 business schools of medicinal materials, 1 school of pharmacology, 1 school of biologicals and 1 health school for the blind. Altogether 854,000 graduated from these schools between 1949 and 1980, 21.6 times more than the pre-liberation figure. The length of schooling ranges from two to three years.

Further Education Further education of health personnel is conducted under the general state policy on education for workers and employees. It is a continuation of secondary and higher medical education. The policy is: To promote in-service education for all health personnel and give prominence to important needs; to draw up overall plans and place the responsibility on organizations at different levels; to carry it out actively within the limits of available resources; and to adopt different forms and emphasize practical results. Eight further education centres have been inaugurated at eight medical colleges. At the provincial level, 21 in-service education colleges for health personnel have re-opened, and centres for further education in specialized subjects have been set up in large hospitals, health and anti-epidemic stations and research institutes. A national network of further education for health personnel has been established: the Ministry of Public Health has the responsibility for the further education of the leading personnel of the provincial public health bureaux, teachers at medical colleges, senior doctors and other senior technical personnel; the provincial public health bureaux are in charge of the further education of the leading personnel of the public health institutions at the prefectural and county levels, of teachers at secondary health schools and at colleges of further education, and of resident doctors; the prefectural and county public health bureaux are responsible for the training of medical and other technical personnel of the commune hospitals and of barefoot doctors. Most further education is offered in the form of study classes lasting from two weeks to a year. A number of people are selected every year to receive further education abroad.

Development of Medical and Pharmaceutical Colleges and Schools

Year	*1949*	*1952*	*1965*	*1980*
No. of medical & pharmaceutical colleges*	22	31	92	109
Enrolment	15,234	24,752	82,861	139,569
No. of secondary medical & pharmaceutical schools	—	320	298	553
Enrolment	15,387	59,407	88,972	244,695

* Not including medical colleges and departments affiliated with universities.

(2) RESEARCH INSTITUTIONS AND PERSONNEL

Before liberation, there were only four medical research institutions in the whole of China, with a staff of less than 300 research personnel. Research departments have gradually increased in number since liberation until a fairly complete research network has taken shape. The 1980 figures show that there were 282 research institutions of Western and Chinese medicine staffed by 18,000 full-time research scientists. These institutions are under the guidance of either the central or local authorities.

The Chinese Academy of Medical Sciences and the Academy of Traditional Chinese Medicine are two of the three national research organizations. The former had in 1980 a research staff of 3,281 scientists, 327 of them were research fellows or associate research fellows. Affiliated with it are five hospitals — the Capital, Ritan, Fuwai and Plastic Surgery hospitals and the hospital affiliated to the Sichuan branch of the Chinese Academy of Medical Sciences, and 20 research institutes specializing in clinical medicine, pre-clinical medicine, plastic surgery, tumour, cardiovasology, epidemiological microbiology, paediatrics, parasitology, dermatology, hygiene, pharmacology, haematology, blood transfusion, antibiotics, virology, medical biology, biomedical engineering, radioactive medicine, experimental animals and medical information. In the past 30 and more years, the Chinese Academy of Medical Sciences has completed 226 research projects.

Affiliated with the Academy of Traditional Chinese Medicine are the Guanganmen and Xiyuan hospitals and the three research institutes of bone-setting, pharmacology and acupuncture and moxibustion. All told, this academy is staffed by 433 research personnel, 47 of whom are research fellows, associate research fellows and veteran doctors. In the 25 years from its founding in 1955 to 1980, the academy has completed 35 research projects.

Local medical research institutes have been set up in 29 provinces, municipalities and autonomous regions. The medical and pharmaceutical colleges and main hospitals, anti-epidemic centres and disease prevention and treatment centres are also engaged in scientific research, participated in by about 6,000 part-time research workers.

The Medical Science Committee of the Ministry of Public Health is composed of over 200 experts and professors of the different branches of medicine. It has 45 sub-committees on special subjects with a total of more than 1,100 members. They are consultative organizations of the Ministry of Public Health.

(3) ACHIEVEMENTS IN SCIENTIFIC RESEARCH

Many successes have been achieved in medical scientific research in the past 30-plus years. Among the many research projects, 335 have won national awards and 802 have received the Ministry of Public Health awards. The following are a few important ones:

Cultivation of Trachoma Virus In 1955, Tang Feifan, director of the Biological Products Institute under the Ministry of Public Health, who died in 1958, collaborated with the department of ophthalmology of Beijing Tongren Hospital and for the first time successfully isolated and cultivated, by means of vaccination of chick embryo, trachoma virus from the conjunctival scrapings of a trachoma patient.

Treatment of Acute Abdominal Conditions and Hepatolith by Chinese-Western Medicine The Dalian Medical College started this method of treatment experimentally in 1958. Simple, economic and easy to popularize, this non-operational method saves the patients from the pains of operations. Its rate of cure is 92.7 per cent in acute abdominal conditions and 64.4 per cent in clearing out stones.

Study of Pain-Suppressing Effect of Acupuncture Chinese physiologists have been studying the reason why acupuncture can stop pain. It became a multi-disciplinary research subject carried out on a nationwide scale since 1965. Prof. Zhang Xiangtong, director of the Institute of Physiology under the Chinese Academy of Sciences, was the first to publish a treatise in 1973, in which he proves on the basis of his experiments that the pain-suppressing effect of acupuncture is brought about by the mutual action and adjustment, in the central nervous system, of the signal delivered by the pricking of the needle and that from the source of pain.

Treatment of Extensive Burns The burns research department of the Shanghai Second People's Hospital has, since 1958, treated 4,407 cases of serious burns and achieved a 91.5 per cent cure rate, which is higher than the international standard. Among those saved was a patient with burns (94 per cent were of third degree) covering 100 per cent of the body surface.

Rejoining Severed Limbs Dr. Chen Zhongwei and his colleagues of the Shanghai Sixth People's Hospital began to rejoin severed limbs in 1963 and have succeeded in 92 per cent of their operations. Between 1966 and 1977, the Shanghai Sixth People's Hospital and Huashan Hospital succeeded in free muscle grafting, transplanting severed limbs after removing the diseased part, remaking a thumb by grafting a toe, and grafting free skin or bones with blood vessels.

Cultivation of Strains of Epithelioid and Fusiform Cells of Nasopharyngeal Carcinoma Many attempts had been made abroad since 1969 to cultivate strains of epithelioid cells of nasopharyngeal carcinoma, but none had succeeded. In August 1975, the Institute of Oncology of the Chinese Academy of Medical Sciences successfully cultivated a strain of epithelioid cells and of fusiform cells of nasopharyngeal carcinoma from the tissue sample of a patient. Both have reproduced extracorporeally for more than 90 generations.

Cure of Chorio-epithelioma Chorio-epithelioma is a grave threat to the health of women. Beginning in 1958, Prof. Song Hongzhao of the department of gynaecology and obstetrics of the Capital Hospital, Beijing, with the assistance of his colleagues, has creatively developed a therapy of early diagnosis and early treatment. So far,

80 per cent of the patients have been saved from immediate death, 35 per cent have survived for more than 10 years, 10 per cent for more than 15 years, and over 100 young patients have given birth to babies after cure. This result is similar to what has been achieved abroad. But Dr. Song's method produces less side-effects.

Early AFP Diagnosis of Liver Cancer In 1978, research fellow Sun Zongtang of the Institute of Oncology under the Academy of Medical Sciences, with the co-operation of other units, employed the method of quantitative evaluation of AFP through radio-rocket electrophoresis with atuoradiography to make early diagnosis of liver cancer. His method, which diagnoses the disease at an early stage when there are not yet symptoms, is more than 98 per cent accurate.

Survey of Common Malignant Tumours This survey, which took three years to complete, was conducted by the tumour prevention and treatment department of the Ministry of Public Health and its counterparts in 29 provinces, municipalities and autonomous regions. Employing the death-tracing method for the first time in China, it revealed the basic laws governing the occurrence and distribution of malignant tumours commonly seen in China. It also shows that cancers of the esophagus, lung and liver are closely related to the local environment and habits of life, and provides the necessary data for the study of cancer prevention.

Artemisia Extract — New Anti-malaria Medicine This new medicine for combating malaria is the outcome of research undertaken by the Institute of Chinese Pharmacology under the Academy of Traditional Chinese Medicine with the co-operation of 19 other units. It is highly and swiftly effective, low in poison-content and applicable for treating cerebral and malignant malaria. Artemisia extract is a new type of compound entirely different in chemical composition from the existing malaria remedies in the world. It follows chloroquine as another break-through in anti-malaria history.

Apart from the above, a number of other important projects have been completed and new advances made in pre-clinical medicine, public health and epidemic prevention, radioactive medicine and clinical medicine (cardiovasology, parasitology, endemiology, ophthalmology, dermatology, infectious diseases, etc.) all of which have promoted the development of medical science and technology.

8. HEALTH INSTITUTIONS AND MEDICAL SERVICES

(1) HEALTH INSTITUTIONS

Administrative Organs Below the Ministry of Public Health in the central government are departments or bureaux of public health at the provincial, municipal and autonomous regional levels; bureaux of public health at the prefectural, autonomous prefectural and provincial city levels; and sections of public health at the county, autonomous county and city district levels. The Ministry of Public Health has departments for medical administration, pharmaceutical administration, traditional Chinese medicine, epidemic prevention, health supervision, health of women and children, medical science and technology, medical education, planning and financial affairs, and foreign relations.

Other Administrative Organizations Related to Ministry of Public Health These include the National

Committee for Patriotic Health Campaign, the State Family Planning Commission and the State General Administrative Bureau of Medicine and Pharmacology. There is also a leading group, set up under the Central Committee of the Chinese Communist Party, for the prevention and treatment of liver fluke in south China. Headquartered in Shanghai, it is led by the First Secretary of the Shanghai Municipal Party Committee and a Vice-Minister of Public Health. Also under the Party Central Committee, the leading group for the prevention and treatment of endemic diseases is headquartered in Shenyang, Liaoning Province, and headed by the First Secretary of the Liaoning Provincial Party Committee and a Vice-Minister of Public Health.

The above organizations are structured independently, each having its subordinate organizations at the provincial, prefectural and county levels. Their executive bodies, however, are generally subordinate to the health administrative departments at the same levels.

Medical and Health Institutions Hospitals, health and anti-epidemic stations, maternity and child clinics, medicine inspection centres, medical and pharmaceutical colleges and schools, and medical research institutions are also set up from the central down to the provincial, prefectural and county levels.

In addition to the medical institutions of the public health departments, some of the industrial and transport departments and the state farms — including their factories — run their own hospitals or clinics. Some also have their own health and anti-epidemic stations, medical colleges and schools and research institutes.

Mass Medical Organizations These organizations include the Chinese Medical Association, All-China Society of Traditional Chinese Medicine, Society of Physiology, Society of Anatomy, Nursing Society, Anti-Tuberculosis Association, Society of Pharmacology, and more than 30 related organizations attached to these societies or associations. They organize academic activities and publish national medical and pharmaceutical journals.

Red Cross Society of China The Red Cross Society of China was founded in 1904 and became a member of the League of Red Cross Societies in 1919. After 1949, it became a member of the executive committee of the League of Red Cross Societies. The Red Cross Society of China was reorganized in 1950 to become a people's health and relief organization of New China, which did much work both at home and abroad. In 1956, the Standing Committee of the National People's Congress ratified the four Geneva conventions revised and signed in August 1949, setting forth protections during time of war for the wounded and sick servicemen in the field, for those wounded or sick at sea, for prisoners of war, and for civilians in time of war.

The Red Cross Society has set up its organizations throughout China. In 1966, there were 25 provincial, municipal and autonomous regional Red Cross societies, over 300 county Red Cross societies and over 50,000 grass-roots organizations, with a total of more than five million members. They helped the public health departments in spreading information about public health, publicizing and organizing first-aid training, family planning, the Patriotic Health Campaign and blood donations. It has done much in disseminating knowledge about medicine and first-aid and protecting the health of the people. In 1966 the national organization of the Red Cross Society was disbanded and all work in the country came to a standstill. The national organization and the local Red Cross societies did not resume work until April 1978. In February 1979, the third congress of the Red Cross Society of China was held in Beijing. The congress elected its council members and standing council members and its president (Qian Xinzhong was re-elected), revised and approved the Regulations of the Red Cross Society of China, and decided on the orientation of its future work.

The Red Cross Society of China has established ties of friendship and co-operation with the Red Cross societies of many other countries. It has sent delegations to many of them on friendly visits or to study medical education and medical services, including blood transfusions. Locating persons and forwarding letters (at the request of someone abroad for someone in China, or vice versa) is a demanding and constant work of the Red Cross Society of China. Entrusted by the Chinese Government, it negotiated with the Red Cross Society of Viet Nam in 1979 on the repatriation of Vietnamese prisoners of war. Giving aid, relief and solicitude to people in distress and refugees abroad is also one of its important tasks. Through its work, it has promoted friendship between the Chinese people and the people of other countries.

(2) MEDICAL SERVICES

Medical institutions at the county level and above are generally operated and financed by the government. Some, however, are operated by collectives. Two-thirds of the rural people's commune hospitals are run by communes, and the rest by the government. The commune-run hospitals receive a fixed amount of subsidies from the government while the rest of the expenses come from funds supplied by the communes and from their own income. The rural co-operative medical service stations or clinics are generally run by the production brigades and participated in by commune members on a voluntary basis. Their premises and plots of land for cultivating medicinal herbs are furnished by the brigades. They are financed by the public welfare funds of the production brigades, money pooled by commune members and their own operational income. The government earmarks a considerable amount of funds every year for financing public health undertakings and subsidizing medical institutions at various levels. Drastic reductions in the prices of medical supplies have been made in the past 30 and more years, the prices of medicines having been cut by a wide margin on six occasions. Contraceptives for family planning and medicines for the prevention and treatment of some endemic diseases are supplied free of charge.

A system of free medical service for workers and employees in cities and towns has been adopted gradually, according to the labour insurance system laid down by the government. The workers and employees pay no insurance fees and, when they fall ill or are injured at work, are given free medical care (including visits to clinics and hospitalization), the expense being shared by the government and the enterprises where they work. In case of injuries suffered on the job, they also receive subsidies for food during hospitalization. Workers and employees who are sick or have suffered injuries at work and women workers and employees during recuperation after childbirth receive different material assistance according to the labour insurance system. Those who have job-related injuries and women workers and employees after childbirth are entitled to full pay.

With the development of the national economy, free medical care has now been extended to the staff and workers at government offices of various levels and cultural, educational and public health institutions, and to all workers and employees of state-owned enterprises (including retirees), officers and soldiers of the Chinese People's Liberation Army, disabled servicemen, and college students. Directly-related family members of workers and employees in state-owned enterprises receive medical subsidies when they are sick.

The government has built a great number of sanatoria and rest homes at scenic spots. Priority in being admitted for recuperation at these places is given to model workers who have made outstanding contributions to the country, and to people who are engaged in work affecting health.

Created by the rural commune members, co-operative medical service is financed mainly out of the public welfare funds of the people's communes and their production brigades. Commune members (including their children) who participate in it pay a nominal amount annually and receive medical care free or partly free according to the circumstances of the commune or brigade. In case of serious illness, the patient is transferred to the commune or county hospital for treatment, with the expenses partly defrayed out of the co-operative medical service fund. To help prevent and treat diseases and train local barefoot doctors and other medical personnel, the medical institutions in the cities and units of the Chinese People's Liberation Army often send mobile medical teams to the countryside and remote frontier areas where conditions are hard.